INSOMNIA

Marina Benjamin is a writer and editor. Her most recent books are *The Middlepause*, *Rocket Dreams*, shortlisted for the Eugene Emme Award, and *Last Days in Babylon*, longlisted for the Wingate Prize. As a journalist, she's written for most of the British broadsheets and served as arts editor at the *New Statesman* and deputy arts editor at the *Evening Standard*. She is currently a senior editor at the digital magazine *Aeon*.

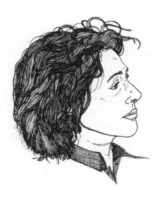

Illustration by Charlie Levy-Sands, child of the author

INSOMNIA

Marina Benjamin

SCRIBE
Melbourne • London

Scribe Publications
2 John St, Clerkenwell, London, WC1N 2ES, United Kingdom
18–20 Edward St, Brunswick, Victoria 3056, Australia

First published in the UK and Australia by Scribe Publications 2018
This edition published 2019
First published in the United States by Catapult 2018

Cover design by Nicole Caputo
Book design by Wah-Ming Chang

Printed and bound in the UK by CPI Group (UK) Ltd, Croydon CR0 4YY

Scribe Publications is committed to the sustainable use of natural resources
and the use of paper products made responsibly from those resources.

9781911344933 (UK edition)
9781925322767 (Australian edition)
9781925693089 (e-book)

Catalogue records for this book are available from the British Library
and the National Library of Australia.

scribepublications.co.uk
scribepublications.com.au

A short, fable-book about long white nights ...
[Benjamin] writes feelingly about the frustrations of being awake
when you don't want to be.' **Zoë Heller, *The New Yorker***

'Anyone who has suffered through the wide-eyed hell
of a sleepless night will find something painfully recognisable
in Marina Benjamin's searingly honest memoir about her years
battling for rest ... *Insomnia* has a dreamlike quality, structured
as a series of fragmented and sometimes unrelated thoughts and
memories ... [There are] moments of stunning poetry, suddenly
interrupted by passages of fevered introspection ... At its heart this
is a book about desire, and the constant dynamic tussle between
hunger and satiation. What does it mean to exist on the
threshold of darkness and light?'
Lucy Hunter Johnston, *Evening Standard*

'An exquisite meditation on time, the dark hours, and the
complexities of longtime love, *Insomnia* is a poetic journey into
the wide-awake, generous, exciting mind of Marina Benjamin.
I couldn't put it down, and my own inner world is richer for it.'
Dani Shapiro, author of *Inheritance*

'Mellow introspection and anecdotal whimsy are spliced
with tidbits of cultural criticism ... Benjamin's is a refreshingly
grounded and sanguine voice.'
Houman Barekat, *The Spectator*

'A sublime view of the treasures and torments to be found
in wakefulness. Entertaining and existential, the brightest
star in this erudite, nocturnal reverie in search of lost sleep,
is the beauty of the writing itself.'
Deborah Levy, author of *Hot Milk*

'Conjuring a spell over those dark hours that threaten to overtake
her, Benjamin's writing, like Scheherazade's fables, manipulates and
even dispels time. One finishes her book as if emerging, ironically,
out of a dream: we cannot say how long it lasted, only that the
sensation will, we hope, stay with us for a while.'
Rajat Singh, *The Rumpus*

'Not so much a lament for lost oblivion as a defiant hymn to the wild
isle of Insomnia.' **Fiona Capp, *Sydney Morning Herald***

'A darkly thrilling beauty of a book ... Benjamin's talent is Arachne-like. The materials she integrates are eclectic, and the resulting constructed web of her thoughts is architecturally robust and resplendent with dazzling prose.'
Tali Lavi, *Australian Book Review*

'As well as a very personal account, it is also a very idiosyncratic cultural history of sleeplessness, a poetic meditation on what we lose and what we gain from these unwilled encounters with brute night. The fragmented structure fits well with the subject, and Benjamin is excellent at describing the jagged loops and whirrs of a mind failing to find rest.' **Ella Walker,** *The Herald*

'Marina Benjamin is the Scheherazade of sleeplessness, spinning tale upon tale, insight upon insight, in frayed and astonishing and finally ecstatic loops.'
Francis Spufford, author of *Golden Hill*

'Benjamin's impassioned and elegant memoir is not just an intimate account of a disorder for which there is still no straightforward cure, but a defiant celebration of its paradoxical potential ... This provocative, at times anguished book has by the end completely overthrown our expectations by repositioning insomnia as a form of resistance, linked to the author's own freedom to create.'
Elizabeth Lowry, *The Guardian*

'*Insomnia* reads with the surreal and suspended cadence of those lonely hours in the night that only the sleep-less experience. It is, therefore, a kind and intimate companion to our meandering, agitated, non-knowing, spiritually naked thoughts at such hours. Keep it by your bedside lamp!'
Sarah Wilson, author of *First, We Make the Beast Beautiful*

'Benjamin writes beautifully. This is a graceful rumination on the "wicked kind of trespass" that is insomnia, a work cogent and allusive as a lucid dream, a palimpsest of insights to dip into, day or night.' **Anna Funder, author of** *Stasiland*

'A really wonderful book — good for night owls too, even if you are not an insomniac. And just for those who are interested in the imagination and creativity.' **Diana Henry**

For Zzz, a sleeper, and
Charlie, intrepid crosser of borders

Who sleeps at night? No one is sleeping.
In the cradle a child is screaming.
An old man sits over his death, and anyone
young enough talks to his love, breathes
into her lips, looks into her eyes.

MARINA TSVETAEVA
'Insomnia'

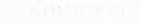

INSOMNIA

Sometimes the rattle of a clapper sounds over your bed. Or a ghostly draft lifts the hairs on the back of your neck, cooling your skin; or there's an upstroke, feather light, along the inside of your forearm. A sudden lurch, maybe just a blink, then a sense of falling upwards and it is there. So are you.

If we insist on defining something in terms of what it annuls then how can we grasp the essence of what is lost when it shows itself? And how can we tell if there is anything to be gained by its presence? This is the trouble with insomnia.

When I am up at night the world takes on a different hue. It is quieter and closer and there are textures of the dark I have begun paying attention to. I register the thickening, sense-dulling darkness that hangs velvety as a pall over deep night, and the green-black tincture you get when moisture charges the atmosphere with static. Then there is the gently shifting penumbra that heralds dawn and feels less like the suggestion of light than a fuzziness around the edges of your perception, as if an optician had clamped a diffusing lens over your eyes then quizzed you about the blurred shapes that dance at the peripheries of your vision. In sleeplessness I have come to understand that there is a taxonomy of darkness to uncover, and with it, a nocturnal literacy we can acquire.

At the velvet end of my insomniac life I am a heavy-footed ghost, moving from one room to another, weary, leaden — there, but also not there. I read for an hour, make myself a cup of tea, and sit with the dog. We stare at each other with big cow eyes and I marvel at his animal knack for sleep. Curling in beside me on the sofa, he is out within minutes, legs splayed like bagpipes, his warm little body rising and falling. If I so much as twitch he snaps awake instantly but without any sense of alarm; he just lifts those liquid brown eyes towards mine, wanting to know if the world is unchanged.

On nights like these I leave a trail of evidence behind me to be discovered and remembered in the morning: my reading glasses upturned on the coffee table, carelessly cast off like a pair of party shoes, an open book facedown on a chair, food crumbs on the kitchen counter. Sapped by fatigue, I stand in the middle of the living room in the dusty light and pull my dressing gown around me. I am trying to puzzle out the clues so as to reconstruct the events of the night before, but I keep blanking. The *mise-en-scène* of morning starts to resemble the scene of a crime. All that is lacking is the body shape outlined on the floor: the missing body, wakeful when it should be sleeping.

There are also luminous moonlit nights, lurid nights, when everything feels heightened and I jerk awake with a fidgety awareness, my mind speeding. In the grip of an enervating mania, I creak my way down the stairs and switch on the computer, scrolling for bad news from places where daylight reigns: an exploding bomb, the wreck of human carnage, floods, fires, terrorist traps. Ordinary disasters. I pace and fret, railing at the dumb news, racing with emotion. I feel held back by the night because I am convinced that the hidden mystery of our beautiful existence might be found in its very bowels. I am looking for insight, for a nugget of value to carry across night's border into morning.

But where is the hidden value in this spinning carousel — a flash memory of my daughter hula-hooping, Earth, Wind & Fire singing 'Ah-li-ah-li-ah', a presentiment of abandonment: am I or am I not loved?

Insomnia (noun): a habitual sleeplessness or inability to sleep. It comes to us from the Latin *insomnis*, meaning without sleep. The insomniac complaint was known to Artemidorus of Daldis, one of the Western world's oldest interpreters of dreams. In his second-century treatise *Oneirocritica*, Artemidorus distinguished mortal dreams that arise out of the dreamer's life experience, and conjure with symbols drawn from the raw materials of his or her desires, from prophetic dreams, or *oneiroi,* which are gifted or sent to us. But the Greeks had another term to denote sleeplessness: *agrypnotic*, from *agrupos*, meaning 'wakeful', which in turn derives from *agrein*, 'to pursue', and *hypnos*, sleep. Insomnia, then, is not just a state of sleeplessness, a matter of negatives. It involves the active pursuit of sleep. It is a state of longing.

What do I long for? I ask myself this question in the witching hours because it cannot be asked by day. On certain turbulent nights this longing is so great and deep and bald it swallows up the world. Defying comprehension, it just is. And I am a black hole, void of substance, greedy with yearning. To be without sleep is to want and be found wanting.

Mostly, though, I long for benevolent Hypnos, dreamiest of the Greek gods, to swoop down over me, scattering his crimson poppies, and drug me into a sweet insentient sleep. Hypnos reminds me that the bestowing of sleep comes from above. It is literally a gift from the gods.

When you cannot get sleep you fall in love with sleep, because desire (thank you, Lacan) is born out of lack. Perhaps there is an inverse relationship here, between the degree of lack and the corresponding degree of love. How much do I love sleep, I wonder. And can sleep love me back? The medieval Islamic poet Rumi seemed to think the relationship might be reciprocal. In 'The Milk of Millennia' he wrote: 'every human being streams at night into the loving nowhere'. I find it comforting to think that we might stream beyond our bedroom walls at night, like a crystalline liquid (or like data), as though our avatars were flowing towards, then alongside those of others in surging formation while our bodies were at rest. I find it reassuring that nowhere can be a loving place. Although when I am revving in the night hours, Nowhere does not feel especially loving.

These days my prime time is 4.15 a.m., a betwixt and between time, neither day nor night. At 4.15 a.m., birds chirrup, foxes scream, and sometimes, when the rotating schedule for landing and take-off from Heathrow Airport collides with my sleeplessness, planes rumble overhead. The quality of the dark is not as pure at this hour as it is earlier. It is porous around the edges. In my bed, I flap and thrash like a grouper caught in the net, victim to an escalating anxiety about the way the darkness appears to be yielding to the idea of retreat. (I don't want it to yield; I want it to last so that I can sleep.) Unable to settle in one position for more than a few beats, I try them all out in turn: the plank, the foetal curl, the stomach-down splat — as if I'd landed on the mattress from a height. Each of these poses is contrived insofar as it corresponds to an idea I have of what relaxation looks like. Some nights I trawl the whole alien repertoire of self-help. I try breathing deeply and slowly like a yogi, my fist pressed into the chakra under my rib cage. I try to stay my galloping pulse, tripped by fretful thoughts I would like to banish, by thinking of water or mountains, or fluffy sheep. I tell myself I am heavy, heavy, heavy. I pursue sleep so hard I become invigorated by the chase.

Through it all, I am aware of a slumbering form beside me, a still mound under the duvet, heaped up like a rock formation under the sky. I peer at the shadow-shaped mass across the bed, my rock, my stay, straining to detect any hint of movement in the dark. Let's call this sleeping form Zzz. I am loath to wake him, knowing that he, like me, is exhausted to the point of defeat. I also know that if my thrashing does wake him he will snarl and shift; occasionally he swipes at me, a big cat in his lair lashing out with a heavy paw. There is a sleep-charged force field around Zzz and woe betide me if I disturb it.

Zzz and I have a history of beds we have slept in together. Hotel beds with silky sheets and too many pillows; beds so old we'd end up rolling into the middle; tufty beds with broken springs in cheap rented flats where we popped corn and watched scary movies through finger fences. In our shared history of sleep there have been beds of character and beds of convenience. Beds that spring out of sofas, supplied by relatives happy to accommodate our long-distance visits, and twin beds (supplied by relatives lacking fold-out options) that create an austere, prohibitive gulf between us, and bring on fits of the giggles. There have been state-of-the-art mattresses we have bought and regretted (especially the orthopaedic kind once believed to be best for backs, but which I now think belong only in jails), and beds we have drooled over on the internet but cannot afford — beds made out of 'memory foam'. We have shared countless beds down the years and across continents, Zzz and me, under mood clouds fair and foul, and we continue to commune by night, in code and often in counterpoise to the way we relate to each other by day.

To share a bed with someone is to entertain a conversation played out in the language of movement and space.

There have been times when this conversation sparkled, I can tell you. Like those weeks we spent in Italy, not long after we first met. I'd been awarded a six-week writing fellowship, which we fattened up with vacation, training south from Milan and Venice, then stopping off in Florence en route to Rome. It was the first time either Zzz or I had seen Italy's golden city. Each day, we wandered ancient twisting streets until our feet hurt, squinting into the sun as we took in architectural triumphs and follies.

We guzzled pastas we'd never heard of, shaped like tiny stars, pigs' tails, and miniature money bags, and ducked in and out of churches, hunting down artworks we had read about in books, before threading our way back to our *pensione* for a daily afternoon nap. Glutted with art, ice cream, and wonder, we slept with limbs entangled, our breathing synchronised, foreheads touching, and when we awoke we had sleepy sex. Such glittering conversations are hard to sustain over time.

You don't need a bed in order to sleep with someone. But the first time I shared a bed with Zzz I was insomniac. At least I refrained from asking him to get up and leave so that I might stand a chance of sleeping, which request had lost me a boyfriend or two in my time. But I suspect that a precedent was set.

Like travel, insomnia is an uprooting experience. You are torn out of sleep like a plant from its native soil, then shaken down so that any clinging vestige of slumber falls away, naked confusion exposed like nerve endings. Sleep, in its turn, is a matter of gravity. It pulls you down, beds you in the earth, burrows you in. In sleep you connect back to the bedrock that provides nourishment and restorative rest.

Rubin Naiman, a psychologist at the University of Arizona's Centre for Integrative Medicine, reminds us that when we turn to sleep aids we often reach for gel-filled eye masks and weighted blankets, to 'swaddling' that acts to counter the restive states of arousal we experience in insomnia. I have noticed that my teenage daughter, in her own struggles with sleep, loads up pillows on top of her head to acquire that longed-for sense of gravity. 'It's not about sleeping on a cloud. It's about sleeping like a stone,' says Naiman.

The body must be grounded to sleep well. I think this is a lesson for the ages. It must be earthed in its own garden bed, or, unmoving, sunk at the bottom of time's river (for when you are asleep time stands still). In her poem 'Sleeping in the Forest', Mary Oliver writes of tumbling into the earth's wondrous embrace, its maternal reclaiming of her, as she falls asleep on the dank and mossy forest floor, slumbering heavily, like a stone on the riverbed. Hypnos would be proud of such a sleeper. Not merely drugged, but comatose.

In the grip of insomnia I am constitutionally inconsolable. Out of humour. It is not just a question of physical disquiet — not just about flapping. Or even existential disquiet (a fish out of water, a plant ripped from the earth), because insomnia is about temperature as well as motion. On nights when I am consumed by the flames of my own thermo-cellular generator, my skin prickles and oozes, the heat radiating off me in waves, the sheets dampening beneath me. If the lights were suddenly to be turned on, I would be glistening. Coated from head to toe by a film of sweat, I would flare red, like a warning.

Ancient physick would most likely designate me a choleric. The basic characteristics of this personality type are hotness and dryness, and its corresponding humour is yellow bile. People of a choleric temperament have appetites that are sharp and quick. Check. They are frequently overcome by ravenous hunger. Check. They are lean and wiry, with prominent veins and tendons. Check. Their metabolism is keen and catabolic, which is to say they generate a lot of heat. Even their urine can be hot and burning. They are prone to anger, impatience, and irritability, but then they are courageous and audacious as well. Check. They are individualists and pioneers who like to lead and to seek out exhilarating experiences. Check. However, their stools tend to a yellowish colour (the bile) and emit a foul odour. Choleric types are notably poor sleepers. Check. Restless at night, they are assailed by indigestion and stress, or by violent dreams that jolt them into states of feverish or fiery readiness.

Fevers notwithstanding, in insomnia it is usually my mind that is on fire. What does a mind on fire look like, I hear you say? Like a Formula One driver tearing up the tarmac. Like a shimmering shoal of restless fish, darting forward together with fleet, quicksilver movements. Like a vacuum cleaner draining juice from the socket and spinning off around the room of its own accord. My insomnia often feels like this: turbocharged. It is not one idea that teases and prods me awake, a finger tickling me in a single spot, wriggling my mind into consciousness. It is as if all the lights in my head had been lit at once, the whole engine coming to life, messages flying, dendrites flowering, synapses whipping snaps of electricity across my brain; and my brain itself, like some phosphorescent free-floating jellyfish of the deep, is luminescent, awake, alive.

In the first book of Proust's *In Search of Lost Time*, Marcel muses on his insomniac experiences, on how he finds himself confused, as if he has been dropped fully conscious but unsuspecting into someone else's waking dream. In his perplexity, he imagines that he has been reading a book about his own life and that his thoughts about himself come second-hand from print; but then he realises that actually he is not in the book but in his bed, and that he cannot separate his recollections from his imaginings. Even so, Marcel can picture an ideal kind of insomnia for himself (the one he yearns for but does not get) in which he wakes at night for just long enough to appreciate the unsullied darkness that envelops him before falling peacefully back to sleep.

The matter of what to do with an overactive brain determined to forge ideas and connections in conditions of sensory blackout troubles me.

I know that the human brain is not a computer and yet computing metaphors are difficult to avoid when what is going on in your night-waking head feels like an electronic event. I'll give you a for-instance. On nights when I cannot easily will myself back to sleep because the switch has already flipped to ON, I begin to sense some unknown part of my brain, some lower-order, engine-room, grafter gland, busy itself running an hours-long system scan. Lucky for me, wakefulness has given me an unexpected window onto its operations. Patiently, systematically, this biological algorithm roots through my store of mental files, searching out broken bits of code — ideas that refuse to link up, shards and stray threads of mental activity — and desperately tries to join them. Then it scans for duplications, thoughts that double up and play over needlessly. All these duplicates and shreds qualify as junk to be cleared out, along with half-formed memories, non sequiturs, ideations stuck in unhelpful configurations, and coiled notions that spiral fruitlessly, going nowhere.

Given that I know that this purging scan is under way, why do I never wake up the next morning feeling mentally refreshed?

The other night, awake again, I began composing a letter in my head to a courier company on the other side of the globe that had failed to deliver a book to me while I was travelling. The company had emailed to say that the driver had not been able to find the (foreign to me, local to him) address. Now, in sleepless monomania, I imagined drafting a letter of quiet fury. In it I would ask why the driver had had such trouble locating the place, when I, a non-native, a mere visitor (and someone with a notoriously bad sense of direction, to boot), had succeeded where they had failed. I would inform the company that other book-delivery services had found the place. That I was staying in a house bursting with publishers, writers, and booksellers, all of them ordering books; that white Jiffy bags had been piling up in the hall and I'd been inspecting them daily, wondering when my book would come. The more solid my case became, the more refinements I thought to add. I felt the courier company ought to know that the book was critical to my research, as well as hard to find second-hand: I had been counting on them! Yet by the time they'd even thought to send up a flare in a last-ditch attempt to reach me I had already been home several days. Never mind that throughout the wakeful working hours of the week that I had kept watch for the book I had never once thought to contact them.

It occurred to me only later that perhaps an additional question ought to be posed — one more pressing than why the book never arrived. The question is this: what if waking life is incapable of adequately attuning us to the needs of our unconscious minds?

Lately I have been experimenting with earplugs to shut up the birds, but beyond the hush they create — the welcome muting of the carnival noise beyond my window — earplugs open up a strange inner world of mysterious echoes and thickening silences. If I listen hard along this internal register I can tune into the dull thud of my heart treadmilling in its cage and sometimes I pick up the coarse whooshing sound of vital fluids sloshing, or wind spiralling through the ammonite tubes of my inner ear. Who knows (and who cares) whether this is just a trick played on us by the senses — an inventive way for the body to fill up the void with something other than nothing. Whatever the cause, it affords us some glimpse into the insomniac's sensorium.

To feel assaulted by the sounds of night is an odd experience for someone like me, who struggles to hear well by day and for whom deafness is part of her genetic destiny. Birds sound like warbling handheld devices. Radiator pipes clang and choke. Water trickles in improbable places I cannot identify. I hear rodents — or bigger — scuttle and scratch as they set up home behind the skirting boards and in the rafters. This reacquaintance with hearing feels like a novelty. It makes me wonder if I will begin to look forward to the orchestrations of the night as I continue to grow harder of hearing.

My father, vain man that he was, flatly refused to wear a hearing aid as he grew deafer and deafer with advancing age. He hated the idea of visibly parading his deficit. But his aversion to hearing aids was, equally, part of his larger refusal of the world; he preferred the atmospheric pressure on the inside of his head just as he preferred the reality screen produced by his own internal projector, throwing up images against every blank wall. My father, the waking dream factory. My mother, now in her mid-eighties, is more profoundly deaf than he ever was. Recently she spent several thousand pounds on an alien-looking apparatus that sits inside her outer ear, invisible to all but the most discerning eye. It sprouts two little antennae over its perforated plastic surface, like a spy device. But it picks up more noise than anything else. I am struck that my parents found such different ways of navigating the world of sound loss, my father judging deafness to be advantageous; my mother giving in to the white noise, losing herself in the buzzing soundscape as the flow of sense washed over her, so that she learned to care more for Being than Meaning.

I would prefer to hear nothing than not enough. In fact, part of me is fast acquiring a taste for the particular kind of sensory numbness that earplugs confer, tuning out the birds while tuning into inner space; stoppering up the world in order to be more attentive to the dark.

Zzz got there long before me. Congenitally deaf in one ear, he hears every sound in mono. Every crash, squeal, thrum, laugh, roar, or — to me — barely audible boom-box bass line from a midnight rave two streets away gets sharpened to a focused pinpoint of sound, penetrating his eardrum like an acupuncture needle. But mono sound is also non-directional: in a world of surround sound, Zzz hears everything as a single-ear assault. When ambushed by loud or intrusive noises he gets confused and defensive, mistaking a slamming car door for an intruder, a smashed bottle in the street for a sally against our barricades. I feel for Zzz in the night-time, when sounds that are merely amplified for me become intolerable for him, not just loud but om-nipresent. By day I am less sympathetic, since I have noticed that deafness, even half-deafness, can be a way to import a bit of contraband sleep into daytime.

Then again, deafness, like sleep, can tune us in to the needs of our unconscious minds.

In Venice's Guggenheim Collection there hangs a painting by the Belgian surrealist René Magritte that speaks to my customary state of mind. It depicts a large lamplit house, partially shrouded by a crop of leafy trees silhouetted in darkness. A pair of upstairs windows glows invitingly, like a pair of mooning eyes, tempting you to picture the comfortable domestic scene unfolding within: children scampering about before bedtime, an elegant woman at her toilette, and because this is a painting from a certain era, some androgynous character in a smoking jacket enjoying a casual cigarette. At first you miss what is disconcerting about the picture. Then, with a creeping sense of becoming alert to a worrying dissonance, you notice that the sky above the shadowy tree line is blue as day and dotted with cotton-wool clouds. The painting, in other words, is bright with contradiction.

Magritte's 'Empire of Light' paintings (there are at least three of them working the same theme) are designed to be profoundly unsettling because they disrupt a fundamental organising principle of life: the categorical separation of night from day. Each brings day and night together into vivid confluence. Nothing is as it should be. Sunlight, ordinarily a source of clarity, causes the kind of confusion and dis-ease we normally associate with darkness, while the insomniac sky serves to intensify the shadow world beneath, making it more inscrutable than ever. The house, in particular — home, haven — is rendered cryptic.

All the time I've laid claim to a home of my own, I have felt as though my body somehow mapped its extent, point to point, as if by a geometry of dotted lines belonging to a pencilled exercise in the art of projection. With its secret corners and lit apertures, its functional zoning, its boundaries and borders that are sometimes open, sometimes closed, my house mirrors my sense of myself as storied and many-chambered, public and also private: a place of ingress and egress. Perhaps when we talk about truly inhabiting a house we are really talking about that feeling of streaming into and around space, dissolving self and other.

In insomnia my sense of tenure can tighten its grip, as I prowl my domain, tracing every lineament of this mutual mapping. But it can also evaporate, as though my mental leasehold on my house had expired. And then, instead of dissolving myself through familiar expanses, contiguous, free-flowing, and at one with my surrounds, I am confronted with features grown suddenly hulking and alien. Everything is transfigured by darkness. Masked in menace.

It sounds crazy but there have been nights when I have felt certain that my house was alive, as though its walls contained a million eyes, and the very fabric of its structure was expanding and contracting around me, inhaling and exhaling me.

Zzz says, 'The other night I dreamt that we would never have sex again.' Then he says: 'When I woke up I thought that I would rather die than shut down so vital a part of myself.' But I have my earplugs in. Perhaps I should tell him that my sense of myself is no longer solid, that I am like a marbled steak that has felt the blade and been finely sliced into feathery slivers. And yet I say nothing. In my inner world, the menopause is coursing through my veins and arteries like a chemical rinse. Another system scan. Allow the program to finish before restarting.

Night is dependent on day, as day is dependent on night. But night and day are yin and yang, north and south, anode and diode. They never appear on the same stage at once, and if they do, as in Magritte's paintings, we are confounded. Except in insomnia, which is a wicked kind of trespass.

The mighty Nyx, Greek goddess of the night and mother of primordial darkness, inhabited a staggeringly sublime abode. Enveloped by blue-black fog, her cave squatted at the edge of the ragged cliff overlooking the bottomless abyss of Tartarus, a place where, as Hesiod describes it, 'the origins and boundaries of everything' are juxtaposed. Twice a day, at dawn and at dusk, Nyx would greet her daughter Hemera, goddess of day, at the door to this cave. They would converse awhile on its ebony balcony, but they never entered the cave at the same time. When one passed out to fly around the world in winged rhapsody, chariot churning up the sky, the other descended into its darkened chambers to wait out her opposite's reign.

As to the rhythm of these comings and goings — its endless replay — we must truly be dolts to believe that every night will be reliably followed by a new day. What if we are wrong? What if we unexpectedly find ourselves stuck in an endless ordeal of night, the dark night of the soul, condemned to a life of perpetual reckoning? Worse, we might be sucked into the eternal night that waits to ensnare us at the end of our days, and from which there is no escape. It seems only fair at this point that I remind you that Thanatos was the brother of Hypnos, and that the relationship between death and sleep might be considered filial. This explains the way death and sleep stand in for each other as metaphors or prefigurings. It also explains why the new light symbolised by dawn is not just an awakening, but a rebirth.

The philosopher David Hume believed we could never know with certainty that a new day will arrive on the coat-tails of night. We can only infer it, based on our uniform experience of their unfailing succession. Yet inference hardly qualifies as watertight reasoning. To put matters as straightforwardly as I can: even a perfectly observed correlation in the world of events — a 100 per cent pairing of this with that — tells us nothing about the mechanisms of cause and effect that might lurk behind the appearance of succession. What is more, when we grasp for those underlying mechanisms we resort to all manner of wild speculation: the hidden hand, a particulate aether, invisible forces and power fields. We imagine finely tuned cosmic mechanisms as intricate as clockwork. But really, who is to say whether one day, in the midst of some almighty huff, the deity might not simply pull the plug on all our celestial tomorrows? And if you live in a spirit-free universe, consider that we might be blindsided by some unscheduled astrophysical calamity that snuffs out the sun like a candle. Either way, that would be that. Eternal darkness. Once and for all time.

Hume knew there were no guarantees underwriting our taken-for-granted diurnal expectations, so he recommended that we make our peace with uncertainty.

We are pretty good at doing this, as it happens. Not just because we are complacent about lazy inference but because we are acquainted with uncertainty by other means. Not least the figure of the absent lover, which is another form of eternal darkness. Take the stoical Penelope, sitting at home in Ithaca, lonesome, bereft, waiting and longing for her husband, Odysseus, to return from the Trojan War. His absence stirs her desire, but then her insomnia curdles that desire into despair. I like to think that Penelope is wide-awake in every sense of the term, aware of her predicament across a range of registers, somatic, psychic, emotional. Yet try as she might, even she cannot penetrate the darkness of not knowing.

When I wish I could do something useful with my fretful nights, I sometimes think of Penelope, who seeks constantly to renew her hope that her missing husband will suddenly reappear. By day, she spends her time weaving a funeral shroud for Odysseus's father, Laertes, fearing that Laertes should not survive were his son to perish before him. But by night Penelope unravels the threads again as a magical act of replenishing her hope. It is true that she also co-opts her sacred funereal task as a cover to deter unwanted suitors jostling to take Odysseus's place by refusing to entertain them until she has completed it. But it is the weaving and unpicking that interests me (not the pretext), for as long as the shroud remains unfinished Penelope can carry on waiting and hoping, suspended in uncertainty, defying death.

The weaving of hopes and fears, dressing up the truth and spinning yarns: this is women's work. So, too, is remembering and forgetting.

Anxiety is women's work as well. I learned how to worry from my mother, for whom anxiety is a proxy for desire: my mother knows she is alive not because she wants but because she worries. Most days she calls me, expressing her concerns. Am I getting enough sleep? Eating properly? Is there sufficient work coming in? When I say yes, yes, and yes again (I mean, why feed her more to stress over), she confides that *she* is not sleeping. Her sciatica is playing up. Do I think she ought to see the doctor? On second thoughts, scrap that. The doctor will only string her along, tell her she's in perfect health and prescribe medication that two days in she will decide to stop taking. The way he's so dismissive of her symptoms — it is beyond a joke. What is more, she says, she is convinced that she has suddenly become allergic to the fish she has taken to buying to whip up easy suppers. Such small-scale anxieties torment her. But my mother's approach to them is wonderfully Kabbalistic: first she names them and so diffuses their power, then she casts them out (mostly onto me) like a rabbi exorcising a dybbuk. Only then can her mind settle. You could say that my mother is temperamentally insomniac.

In her marriage, my mother bore the full burden of anxiety, whereas my father, like a child, worried about nothing. She made it her job to anticipate his every need before he recognised, much less named them, and in this way he retained a kind of willed innocence throughout the fifty-odd years they spent together. My mother provided meals, transport, cash management, affection, emotional support, social distractions, and commonsense solutions to their various material problems, while my father simply floated — *sleepwalked* — through the world from day to day, inferring the bounty would last. This kind of trade-off is part of the unequal exchange of marriage.

Curious to know if it is possible to sleepwalk by day, I look it up. And in theory it is, if you accept that the essence of sleepwalking consists in the shutting down of certain parts of the brain that generate conscious awareness of a person's actions and surroundings. In sleepwalking, the 'emotional brain', governed by the primitive limbic system, is active. So, too, is the dumb but tremendously effective motor system. What is switched off is the 'rational brain'. It follows from this that sleepwalkers might just be insufficiently vigilant.

Penelope's marriage, like so many templates handed down to us, written in stone, likewise skews unequally. Odysseus unquestionably gets to be the hero of the piece. Larger than life, more idol than man, he fights wars, travels the world, and beds nymphs, while Penelope simply frets. That is to say, she battles the darkness of his absence in her insomnia. Oh, and there are frets in weaving as well.

It seems unfair. Doesn't Penelope qualify as valiant, too? Actively, vigorously, she rejects one suitor after another: suitors who keep coming at her like armed soldiers crawling out of enemy trenches; suitors who would usurp her beloved, drink from his cup, wear his mantle, and sleep in his bed. Against this menace Penelope's resolve is practically superhuman. Especially when you consider that she has been abandoned in Ithaca for twenty years and that the suitors paying her court are half her age (which is surely somewhat tempting). Also, there are legions of them: 108 according to Telemachus (tittle-tattling on his mother), but one scholar I've read counts 191. I would like to allow that the long-suffering and faithful Penelope is heroic in her own way, for she is defiant, self-denying, determined, and capable of enduring great hardship and sorrow. It is not my kind of heroism, that is for sure, but the alternative is deeply unpalatable. Most critics of classical literature fix on the shroud that never gets finished to insist that Penelope's chief quality is wiliness or cunning. In their book, she is just another woman who weaves lies.

I want to say more about insomnia and love, in that both are states of being that pitch us face-to-face with a stinging absence. In insomnia, we crave oblivion — that escape from consciousness, which sleep appears to confer on everyone but us — and in so doing we reaffirm our uneasy relationship to the world of material necessity. Lovers, meanwhile, assert their fealty against the complete absence of any certainty about the future, as though love were a concrete thing that might be thwacked ahead of ourselves like a hockey puck to stake a claim on new ground.

'Love like sleep requires immeasurable trust, a fall into the unknowing,' says one scholar of sleeplessness. But let's bring the two into more intimate proximity. In insomnia we encounter the very heart of love's darkness: the essential otherness of the beloved.

When Zzz and I began regularly sharing a bed together after that first restive night, our sleep dovetailed into perfect accord. It was harmonious. We were like the ancient landmass of Pangea, fused into a single state of being. But then, slowly, incrementally, a continental drift set in and we began to separate bodily, imperceptibly at first — one complaining of overheating, the other of needing their own pillow — and before we knew it, each of us, me and Zzz, had become continents in our own right: miniature tectonic entities, separated by a swathe of night.

Every now and then, I steal a look at Zzz's sleeping form, melding into the blackness of the night, blended into virtual immateriality, and I long to buy a ticket to sail over to his continent, away from Snore Awake and Restive Tossing and across to the land of Peaceful Slumber. Intrepid explorer that I am, I would brave the choppiest waters to get there. Willingly would I fall into unknowingness, becoming blind to my faltering steps; gladly would I forfeit my understanding. All it would take is for me to proffer an outstretched hand.

It's so simple a tender. Yet you'd be astonished at how regularly I stumble before its prospect: unable to relax into the companionability of night, I am forced to patrol my own borders. It is as if my will has been impounded. Clamped and bound according to the dictates of some higher-order bureaucratic lockdown. The maddening frustration of it recalls those rare and panicked states of sleep when you are awake enough to know a mosquito is buzzing in your ear but you are incapable of swatting at it because a crushing bodily paralysis, pushing down on every part of you, pinning you to your bed, flatly forbids it. The wrong bit of you is sleeping, the wrong bit awake. In such a state it is all too easy to flip out, to feel your head become a pressure pot; your panicky resolve, the steam jiggling its lid from within. Your command and control centre is embroiled in internal conflict. To crown it all, for all those agonising minutes spent fluttering in the bell jar, the oxygen of free will draining steadily away, you are at that goddamn insect's blood-sucking mercy.

This is the closest any healthy human being can come to experiencing 'locked-in syndrome' — that abominable state of imprisonment (an island within an island) which the late French journalist Jean-Dominique Bauby was forced to endure following a stroke, and that he wrote about in *The Diving Bell and the Butterfly*. I say wrote, but, in fact, with infinite patience, he dictated the book to a scribe, letter by letter, by moving his eyeball (the only part of his body he could command) whenever she alighted with a pointer on the character he wished to use. Mercifully, not long after completing his testimony — a paean not to suffering, but to love and the richness of life — death arrived to release him from the exquisite torture of being locked in.

4.22 a.m. Now I come to think of it, it has been a recurring trait in my insomniac experience to embark on insect-killing sprees. Slipper in hand, I slap at this or that crawling, buzzing, or creeping thing: a housefly that is already half-dead and stirred into life only by its proximity to my warm body — another living, breathing form — and for which a good wallop with a slipper seems a fitting kind of fate; recently, and memorably, in Spain, an odd-looking flattish centipede, which a quick search on the internet revealed was 'the biting kind'. Yet it squished so easily underfoot, its body releasing a colourless watery fluid and all its legs detaching into floating V-shaped filaments. The creature literally melted away, like a bad dream.

Problem #1. Insomnia makes an island of you. It is, bottom line, a condition of profound loneliness. And not even a dignified loneliness, because in insomnia you are cannibalised by your own gnawing thoughts.

Problem #2. On balance, I would rather be an island than have to endure some landlocked state of being, lacking in boundaries and natural definition. I would rather be a landmass unto myself, a sanctuary. And once I get there, please don't go messing up my solitude.

From the depths of the benign darkness I call velvet, I often wonder at all the other unseen insomniacs twisting awake in their own beds, across street and town, nation and globe — beacons to my beacon. Individually, we are like those luminous dots on an epidemiologist's map, discrete pinpoints of consciousness, suffering in isolation, our minds powering away while covering as little fruitful distance as a runner pounding out meaningless kilometres in the gym. Imprisoned within these solitary cells of wakefulness, insomniacs make for a strange kind of collective. We possess geographical presence — which carries its own weight. We boast blustery swatches of global coverage, dense regional clusters and inexplicable but nonetheless wired outliers: we own statistical relevance. No doubt we could easily spew a textbookful of shared anxieties. Yet we cannot commune with one another.

Some kind of party, this. The incongruity of it clearly impressed itself on Charles Simic, who in his poem 'The Congress of the Insomniacs' pictures insomnia as a vast but empty ballroom. Its ceiling is gilded and its walls mirrored; there is an usher with a flashlight, someone is to deliver a no-doubt starry address, and, Simic trills, 'everyone is invited'.

Simic's doomed congress depresses me. But what other collective noun might we propose as an alternative? A brightness of insomniacs? A flare? A fret?

The sleepless constitute an unlikely population, to be sure, and yet most reports insist we are a growing one. It is as if the human body has been forgetting in near epidemic proportions how to perform a taken-for-granted task, like breathing or digesting, or producing hormones.

(Our global swatch on the epidemiologist's map is spreading like a forest fire.) This sleep deficit affronts us, much as would a theft, because unlike our historic forebears, accustomed to snatching their rest in irregular bursts, often wherever they could lay their heads, we moderns feel entitled to one long, continuous dive into insentience. With work infiltrating every realm of our private lives we tell ourselves that we have at least earned that much. Yet despite having accorded sleep a privileged space — a room of its own, the kingly bedroom, furnished with darkness and quiet, goose-down duvets and high-tech mattresses — Hypnos continues to taunt and elude us.

Perhaps we should think harder about this contradiction as we lie restless and awake, islanded in our beds, staring at the ceiling.

The island. Lonely land of 'I'. Sometimes I think there is no better metaphor for despair, for the feeling of being shored up behind your own defences, cut off from the larger part of humanity and with nothing but your looping dark thoughts for company. In insomnia, my island self floats alone in a sea of night, my bed a sturdy raft, darkness lapping at my shores. Zzz is next to me, but miles away. In those lonesome hours when I fear I might drown in a well of unspecified longing, I sense a danger that my most intimate space might also become my most alienated. Estranged from the night, I am locked out of my own rest. If I reached out to Zzz would I even find him?

I go back and forth over the virtues of island life, unable quite to shake off a romance that has been with me since childhood. A romance that found its worthy idol in Robinson Crusoe. I first came across the Crusoe story watching an old black-and-white, and (I believe) French-made, television serialisation that I realised later was remarkably faithful to Daniel Defoe's novel. It was broadcast every Saturday morning as part of an energy-packed diet of children's programming, and even now I can summon the plangent strains of its theme tune, played on violins. The series arrived on our screens when I was too young to have encountered despair. But I *was* old enough to recognise resilience and I saw its fingerprint everywhere: in Crusoe's daily ritual of carving a notch on a piece of wood — a measured action that seemed to evince nothing less than a mastery of time; in his building enclosures for rearing goats; and in his determination to stay dry whenever besieged by tropical storms, when he would hunker down under a jury-rigged canopy made of palm fronds.

Each week I could barely wait to discover what new-fangled invention this TV Robinson would devise to nudge his tree house (already rather stylish, in a cane-strewn, island-chic kind of way) into an ever closer approximation of civilised comfort: a pulley-operated ceiling fan fashioned by twisting old vines into rope; a fully stocked bar, complete with brandy and crystal glassware filched from his own wrecked ship. I was completely sold on the idea that if only Robinson could build a good-enough replica of the world he had left behind him then he would cease to hanker after rescue. All that was required of him emotionally, I believed when I was ten, was a bit of fortitude. Now I know that one needs a complete toolkit of emotional equipment to build something out of nothing.

Defoe wrote his story amid the heyday of a new mercantile age, working via its simple premise (man marooned, man survives) through every motif that would come to characterise the Enlightenment. Crusoe is the lone white crusader, transporting civilisation with him wherever he goes, even unto the ends of the world, where he comes face-to-face with himself, alone. He cultivates the wild with missionary zeal and brings order to chaos. He is industrious, indefatigable, and ingenious. What keeps him awake at night are productive thoughts about what he might make, or do next, or record in his diary the day following. Crusoe does not merely pass the time: he positively consumes it.

Robinson Crusoe (1719) came on the heels of a century-long campaign that saw Dutch, English, French, Portuguese, and Spanish merchant ships colonise faraway lands for trade, exporting gunpowder and measles in exchange for sugar, coffee, and gold. In many ways the novel models that century. Defoe's fictional hero echoes the European trader's conquistadorial sense of himself as the light in the darkness, and he contains within him all the other 'good' qualities that Enlightenment thinkers set in opposition, one against the other, as if at war: consciousness versus the unconscious, day versus night, magic versus reason, and wakefulness versus sleepy ignorance. In Defoe's novel that quality of dopey ignorance resides in Friday, the savage whom Crusoe takes under his wing and educates. But in reality this sleepiness of mind was embodied in the figure of the slave.

The sorry truth (and guilty secret) behind European civilisation — the unimaginable wealth it accrued to itself! — is that it was purchased on the back of a vast colonial machinery that systematically invaded the 'dark continents' and enslaved their peoples, creating an international economy built on enforced labour. The entire enterprise rested on the premise that the black body was unquestionably inferior, both ignorant *and* expendable; and this so-called ignorance was understood as having kept black people in a kind of perpetual night. But there is a doubling down of darkness involved in this equation, more unforgiveable still, in that the brutalities of slavery were carefully hidden from a growing consumer class back home in Europe, so dazzled by the brilliance of sugar, its medicinal qualities, its ability to preserve foods and ferment alcohol, not least the sheer sweet delight of its crystalline granules, melting on the tongue, that it could no longer see.

Surely it is no coincidence that the money-spinning products extracted from distant lands to feed the expanding economies of Europe were stimulants, one and all? Tobacco, coffee, sugar: generators of mass insomnia.

As it happens, I gave up tobacco long ago (nineteen years, but who's counting) and I can go for long, intermittent stretches without caffeine. But sugar is another story. I will accept it in any form, powder, liquid, granular, solid. I would take the stuff intravenously were it

on offer outside a hospital. Plus I have never met a pud-
ding that I did not like — not a custard, fool, tart, or
ice cream, not a cake, junket, jam, pie, trifle, syllabub,
nougat, brittle, or taffy. And once I have begun, I do not
stop. Zzz says that when it comes to me and cake it is a
case of death by a thousand slices. In my defence I can
only say that, like everyone else, I have been *taught* to
like sugar.

In *Sweetness and Power*, the economic historian Sidney
Mintz traces the growth of the sugar trade. He explains
how sugar was actively pushed on consumers, begin-
ning with the English, where 'sugar [was] pumped
into every crevice of their diet'. The French followed
suit and, after them, the Americans. Mind-boggling
profit was to be gained from the sale of sugar; and
the cheaper it got, morphing over time from luxury
commodity into everyday necessity, the more of it we
consumed.

Mintz quotes an English teacher visiting the 'sugar island' of Barbados in 1645, a half-century before Defoe
published *Robinson Crusoe*, who just about puts it in
nutshell form. Barbadian plantation owners, he says,
had purchased 'no less than a thousand negroes' from

slavers over that twelve-month season alone: 'in a year and a halfe they will earn with God's blessing as much as they cost'.

I have talked about the darkness of not knowing, but what about the darkness of not wanting to know? The darkness of blinkered ignorance. This is the sleep that the slave traders, plantation owners, merchant ship owners, and wealthy investors back home (who exerted themselves only in extending credit) counted upon engendering among their countrymen and women in order to propagate their trade abroad, unchecked.

Most consumers today recognise that capitalism has its dark side (we have all read our pocket Marx). We know about the alienation that results from severing the workforce from the means of production — from land, tools, raw materials, and craft. We know about exploited child workers, sweatshops, and zero-hour contracts. Yet slavery is far darker than capitalism, for in slavery the black body is *part* of the means of production, a tool or instrument in and of itself. Slaves, you see, have nothing to sell: not even their labour. Instead, like the commodities they produce, they, too, are bought, sold, and traded.

Women have a better cultural understanding of this exchange than men do. They know what it means when their bodies and their labour represent an unacknowledged capital asset. What is more, women grasp the essence of standing as surety against risk: the risk of love foundering, the risk of not being seen, the risk of not managing to achieve oneself.

Still, you could say that the evils inflicted upon faraway lands and peoples by the colonial merchant traders of the seventeenth and eighteenth centuries eventually came back to plague us. Marx summed it up with characteristic bite when he complained that the capitalist production that fuelled the voracious new markets of the industrialised nineteenth century 'grafted the civilised horrors of overwork, onto the barbarous horrors of serfdom and slavery'. Marx might have added that as we in the West became slaves ourselves, to the clock, the market, the railroad (and later, motorway) — to capitalised production itself — it became necessary to consume ever greater quantities of sugar, tobacco, and coffee, if only to stay awake through the long days and nights given up to oiling the gears of the monstrous machine. And so the wheel turned.

One of the things I love about Zzz is that the older he gets, the more radical he becomes. Much of the time he is too traumatised by world events to bear reading about them: he feels undermined by news the way bodily fatigue undermines me. But then he girds himself and dives in, tanking up on commentary and analyses, because, as he tells me, knowledge is power. To be forewarned is to be forearmed, and all that. I no longer believe that knowledge is power (I mean, just look at the world and its idiot-king leaders). But I do think that knowledge can pave the road to resistance.

Zzz hates people who insist that enjoying material sufficiency only makes you more avaricious. To spite them, and to make a stand for an alternate morality, he is lavish in his own way, to the point of being profligate. Tirelessly, he spends himself helping out voluntary organisations — schools, literary development agencies, local theatre companies, our teenager's music camp, the neighbourhood hospice — and he regularly gives away his money to people who have less than he does. His generosity is reparative. It is his rearguard fight against the money-worship that breeds injustice and inequality. Zzz's postcolonial conscience is clean. Perhaps that is why he sleeps so well.

One afternoon, a few years back, an Iranian woman knocked at our door. Zzz happened to be home. She told him about her life in Iran and her attempts to defend her sectarian values against the totalitarian Islamic regime. She and her husband were educated people; they believed in religious pluralism and tolerance and saw no need for different faith groups to shout threats and throw rotten vegetables at each other from across the picket line. Her husband and comrade in arms had been arrested, branded an enemy of the state, and thrown into jail for his troubles. The woman showed Zzz pictures of him squaring up to the camera with defiant eyes, his lips a firm line beneath his bristly black moustache. She wept. Zzz invited her into our home, made her Turkish coffee, and pledged to help. He donated a generous sum to the woman's campaign to get her husband released. A year or so later she returned. Her husband was still in jail.

There is a poem that I should love to share with Zzz, for no other reason than that it would delight him. Elizabeth Bishop's 'Crusoe in England' offers a poetic reimagining of Defoe's story set on an island that is the very antithesis of paradise. Let us be clear. There are no sandy white beaches lined with swaying palms here: no fruiting shrubs or singing birds, no colourful array of tropical flora, and no ship-rescued booty. Crater-pocked, ashen, and largely barren, Bishop's island is a rainy 'cloud-dump', smelling of 'goat and guano'.

Bishop's Crusoe, meanwhile, is a self-pitying dullard who, when not drunk, spends a good deal of his island life dangling his legs over the mouth of a spent crater, counting dead volcanoes. This shitty, sterile island has only one kind of everything: one kind of goat, one kind of turtle, one snail, one man, and one burning sun. There is also only one kind of berry, dark red and sour-tasting, with which Crusoe makes the stinging brew that goes straight to his head. Once intoxicated, he 'whoops and dances', playing his homemade flute and prancing among the goats like a crazed fawn. Sober again, he sinks back into his 'miserable philosophy' — the very opposite of enlightened.

Overwhelmed by a sense of his own inner poverty, this Robinson is unable to bestow civilised values on anything. He berates himself for his inadequate education, for not knowing enough Greek or astronomy, and for only half-remembering the poems he once learned by heart, at school. He is shamed by his deficiencies. Boredom eats at him. He is tired of goats bleating, gulls shrieking, and turtles hissing. One day, to relieve the monotony, he dyes one of the goats berry-red, but then its mother refuses to recognise it. When Friday finally shows up, this Robinson laments that his savage companion is not a woman (another lack, another sterility). Eventually the island gets so deep under his skin, it enters his bloodstream. Nightmares haunt his sleep:

nightmares of other islands
stretching away from mine, infinities
of islands, islands spawning islands,
like frogs' eggs turning into polliwogs
of islands . . .

Bishop's poem contains a lesson that ought to knock my island-ideal off its pedestal once and for all. The lesson is this: islands can only beget islands. The insomnia that afflicts her Crusoe is toxic.

Zzz says, 'I wish you would go and see the doctor again,' when I complain that my eyes are stinging from lack of sleep and that my brain feels spongy, as though waterlogged. I want to cry all the time, for no evident reason.

'She'll give you something strong to break the cycle and change up your rhythms,' he says.

'But then I'll just become a zombie,' I tell him, and raise my arms out in front of me to take zombie lunges at him at in the kitchen.

'Better a zombie than a ghost,' he says.

He does not say: *because at least a zombie is present*. But this is what he means.

When Zzz is in a mood to reminisce about when we met, it is a quality of electric presence he likes to recall, a sense of being alive and loving life, and being there and being real: a mass of blood and guts and knotty desires. Romance, especially the chemical kind, is like that, a living thing. But factor time into that equation and the variables involved need to be realigned. You have to allow that life's most ordinary demands, applied day by day, can smooth the textural interest of the most durable of bonds. Even those forged in commonalities so deep they are subterranean. Foundational.

I am saying that the electricity can stop sending sparks through you. In my experience this is a matter of amplitude, however, not supply. We are still on-grid, Zzz and I, still connected to the the mains.

Even so, Zzz says that nowadays I am present mostly in my writing, by which he means I am present only to myself. I don't say it out loud, but insomnia, too, is manifestly about presence.

In truth I am already a zombie. My skin is crawling with discomfort, as though some werewolf form lurking within wants to split it open and burst free. My head lolls with the effort of keeping myself upright. My eyes are glassed over. I am out of sorts with my self. My lack of intent turns me into an alien blob, a sack of seething pulp. I am hungry for whatever it is that makes us human.

It goes without saying that I know all about sleep aids, because insomnia and I have history. Bound together so tight we've experienced all the phases of love, from thrill to bewilderment to boredom and back again. Like the phases of the moon. Insomnia is the thief of my repose and demon lover both. Moonstruck by wakefulness, I have many times looked to sleep aids for succour and I have burned through varietals galore, most of which worked in brief, hopeful spurts, before flatlining.

Ranked in no particular order, these include:

i) Catnip for humans, otherwise known as vale-
rian root. Bought across the counter from any
herbalist, also health stores with aspirations.
You brew it into a tea to drink before bedtime
then hope against hope.

ii) At the other end of the scale, temazepam and
its cousins. I have practically begged for these
rhomboid beauties from stony-faced doctors
who make a virtue of prescribing only a dozen
or so every few months. For your own good,
they explain: to stop you getting addicted. More
recently, with my phasic insomnia now a relent-
less nag, I've taken a non-benzodiazepine hyp-
notic agent called zopiclone. It puts you to sleep
for six or seven hours straight, but the next day
it's as if a cat pissed in your mouth.

iii) Meditation. Actually, I pretty much gave up on
this before I started, terrified of the blankness I
imagined it led to.

iv) Nytol. One of a range of antihistamine prepa-
rations that I have dabbled with, and a current
favourite. But should I take the 'One-a-Night'
or 'Two-a-Night' kind? It is difficult to know.
The dilemma here has been discovering that
the Two-a-Night kind is not worth buying: the

multiple is there only to fool you, since even two of them are weaker than the other sort, the One-a-Night. Besides, if you can take two a night, why not experiment with taking two of the One-a-Night tablets? That's my feeling, anyhow.

Rubin Naiman, who is not a witch doctor but a sleep doctor, bemoans the way that 'sleep has been transformed from a deeply personal experience to a physiological process; from the mythical to the medical; and from the romantic to the marketable'. This is why there exists a whole booming economy obsessed with sleep metrics and insomnia cures, all of it hokey. For, as Naiman so rightly points out, 'sleeping pills produce a kind of counterfeit slumber by inducing amnesia for night-time wakefulness. They do not heal insomnia; they suppress its symptoms.'

Besides, you never wake from an opioid sleep or antihistamine-induced slumber feeling rested. You wake up feeling heavy-limbed, lug-headed, one-dimensional. Sleep aids such as these do not simply fail to heal insomnia: they exchange one ailment for another.

You would think that writing on insomnia has turned me into some kind of expert! Practically everyone I meet now tells me about their sleep troubles. It often turns out to be one of those earplug moments, since there is barely a story I have not heard, a pill I've not tried, or a method I haven't worked before. But it is the mathematics of insomnia that really kills me: the never-ending count of hours lost and gained logged in the ledger of sleep missed and unexpectedly found that every insomniac carries in their head as an account of their own sorry deficiency. Perhaps, after all, the collective noun that fits us best is a *calculation* of insomniacs.

One of my friends told me how she scissors pictures from glossy magazines of imposing king-size beds topped with fluffed-up pillows, spread with thick duvets and quilted coverlets, and with swags of material draped over everything to conjure the requisite degree of swaddle. Made of rich damasks, pima cottons, jacquards and silk, this bedding is designed to soothe and cajole, lull and coddle, enticing sleep. It calls out to her. Whenever my friend is sleepless, she pulls out her stash of soft-furnishings porn and projects herself into the frame.

Most prized among this collection of hers are pictures she has snipped from brochures advertising cruises, so that as well as imagining herself sinking into the comfort of a bed in a luxury yacht, with views stretching out over moonlit horizons, glinting dark off the water, she can, at least in her head, feel the gentle rock of the boat and listen to the waves tugging at her from beyond the porthole of her womb-like berth. This, too, is swaddling.

Then there is the fellow insomniac who introduced me to skullcap. You have not slept until you have tried skullcap.

Skullcap is a plant and it goes by many other beautiful names: blue pimpernel, *Scutellaria*, Grand Toque, helmet flower, hoodwort, mad-dog herb, mad-dog skullcap, mad weed, Quaker bonnet, and *scutellaire*. It should be taken with caution because it can damage the liver, but then so can alcohol, which I happen to be both wanton and incautious in consuming — often in combination with sleep aids. But when you are desperate, and your skin is crawling and your eyes bulging and your head dropping and your brain itching, and you cannot get warm and you cannot be still, then you will reach for skullcap. And, believe me, when you take skullcap you will sleep the proverbial sleep of the dead.

My mother slept under the stars as a child. Imagine that. On impossibly hot Baghdad nights, her entire family dragged thin mattresses upstairs to replicate on the rooftop of their high-walled town house in the Old City the very same arrangements of privacy they enjoyed in their bedrooms. Each couple had its allocated space, curtained off from the extended family by sheets suspended as screens. My mother and her sister shared a cozy corner cubicle, where they were treated to the sounds of the street drifting up to them, mangled and hazy. This kind of sleeping, sleeping that is essentially collective, dormitory-style, is reassuring. It evens out the odds on insomnia. If you are awake, it is more likely that someone else will be too.

But my mother does not recall nights of agitation and turmoil. What she remembers is wriggling beneath the sheets, chattery with excitement, trading whispered secrets with her sister under the sky's glittering blanket. Then, when the gossip ran out, the two of them would gaze up with lump-in-throat wonder at the star-spangled magic in motion. What can it be like to have the sky for a ceiling and the soft breeze for walls? To have the rooftop for a floor and the desert wind blowing welcome dreams your way? It must feel like pumicing the deadening surface right off your existence and exposing raw skin to the air.

I, too, long to be taken out of myself, to feel enlarged by contemplating the grandness of the vaulting heavens above. It isn't angels I wish to see, nor sprites and fairies, not winking stars or alien ships: it is the impossible vastness of the cosmos itself, the infinite depths of its receding darkness — Rumi's 'loving nowhere' — that I long to reach out to and to touch.

The French philosopher Gaston Bachelard has probed the unlikely relationship between outer immensity and inner intensity — the one cool and distant, the other hot and insistent. In *The Poetics of Space*, a fat coffer of a book, rich with insights coined like silver and gold, he pictured this relationship as intimate, as if the trusting act of opening up the soul might allow us to gobble up the whole of creation. Somehow, in Bachelard's calculation, the body is capable of becoming a vessel for containing the world. Which is what love feels like, too, is it not: astonishing in its expansiveness?

It is almost too much for one person to bear, this feeling of cosmic aggrandisement — this sense that by contemplating the heavens one becomes not just spiritually enlarged, but spookily attuned to every possible and as yet unrealised potential, as if channelling time itself. Anything, it seems, could happen.

In my heightened, near-euphoric states of sleeplessness, I can count a handful of memorable occasions when I have felt this way, porous as the night itself, open to whatever might come my way and at one with the fluid universe. Most of the time, though, the very opposite is true. I feel contracted in insomnia, hemmed into my own head and oppressed by the impenetrable dark. My bedroom is like an oven awaiting the igniting flame: a dead space.

When insomnia strikes in night's viscid and inky depths the limits of your vision are all too palpable. You feel occluded by darkness; pressed into your bed, all your horizons are obliterated. It is suffocating, this oppression.

Vladimir Nabokov once likened insomnia to a solar flare (the word he used was *sunburst*) because he loved the way that sleeplessness left him feeling 'joggy, jittery and buzzy'. All the same, he dreaded absolute darkness and insisted upon leaving his bedroom door slightly ajar at night, saying: 'Its vertical line of meek light was something I could cling to, since in absolute darkness my head would swim, just as the soul dissolves in the blackness of sleep.'

Too often what keeps me awake these days is pain, which is another form of contraction. The pain is concentrated in my hip, from where, like the central blip on a radar screen, it pulses steadily, and every now and then it sends rods of fire down one of my legs. This is the kind of pain that demands attention, eats up my focus. Lying awake, it is as if all of my body, invisible in the dark, has become my hip, as if I am morphing under the covers into some Picasso-like woman, every part of me reconfigured into twisted joints articulating around magnified nodes of discomfort.

And so I get up. I get up to escape the pain, and to free myself from sweats both hot and cold (the whole menopausal caboodle) and to prevent myself grinding my teeth, a largely unconscious activity that, over time, has worn down my front three bottom teeth to chalky stumps, dentine exposed along their top ridges like a seam of precious ore in a craggy rock. Some nights my jaw throbs from the grinding, a pounding ache such as you get when the dentist is fumbling too long inside your mouth, bashing and pulling at your molars. When I move about, the pain recedes, gets supplanted by other sensations — and so I get up.

When I cannot surrender myself to sleep this is how I broker a truce with wakefulness.

Yet what would I not give for a spell of enchanted sleep, a dreamless, inert, and benign slumber such as the stuff that fairy tales are made of? I'm talking about pinpricks, hexes, and poisoned-apple territory, those thorny gateways to a somnolent paradise. Not sugar and spice and all things nice, which only keep you awake.

Paradox #1. As every insomniac knows, the more you try to will yourself to sleep, the more sleep will evade you. The push-me-pull-you logic underlying the problem is easily explained, since it is impossible to strive at yielding or to actively prepare oneself for passivity. As William Wordsworth (sounding sorely tested) complained in his ode 'To Sleep':

Even thus last night, and two nights more I lay,
And could not win thee, Sleep! by any stealth:

Painful experience has taught Wordsworth that you cannot trick yourself into sleep, nor gain it by virtue of being deserving: you cannot wheedle or inveigle when it comes to oblivion! And you cannot command sleep either, any more than you can command the elements. Sleep is predicated on submission. It will not be bidden, only beckoned, as Wordsworth himself eventually learns. 'Come,' he intones.

Paradox #2. Sleep is in any case perverse. Invite it over and it will spurn you, deny it and it ambushes you. Our relationship with sleep is fundamentally embattled.

Gilgamesh, wayward warrior-king of ancient Uruk (my ancestral homeland), is one of literature's great insomniacs, locked out of sleep by a sweeping exultation over the many battles he has won and the multitudes of lives he has taken. Gilgamesh prowls through the epic prose-poem that bears his name like a hungry hyena, his anxious wakeful mind always second-guessing itself, never satisfied, always wanting more (land, wealth, women, blood). Insomnia is greedy, after all. It is also, in Gilgamesh's estimate, a triumph: not for him the darkness of mortality. For him there is only the light of the everlasting vigil — the eternal watch for enemies — and an appetite for battle, which, in turn, precludes sleep. You might say that Gilgamesh is at war with himself. That his real battlefield is the battlefield of the mind.

In *The Epic of Gilgamesh*, insomnia stands in for ambition: and Gilgamesh's ambition is boundless, which is to say that it respects no borders, neither territorial nor diurnal. In Gilgamesh's reckoning mortality itself is just another threshold. He longs to be immortal, like Utnapishtim — a Mesopotamian Noah figure gifted with everlasting life by remorseful gods who send a flood to kill humankind and all too nearly succeed. Utnapishtim duly puts Gilgamesh to the test and commands him not to sleep 'for six days and seven nights'. Only then does sleep come, uninvited and unwanted like the contrarian that it is, and sink our prickly hero into a deep and all-too-human slumber.

While we are on the subject of perversity, I should tell you that I recently signed up to a five-week course of cognitive behavioural therapy (CBT) aimed at curbing my insomnia. Instantly I have begun to sleep as never before. It's like booking an appointment to see the doctor only to find that your vexing symptoms suddenly disappear.

Towards the end of 1906, two French scientists, René Legendre and Henri Piéron, performed a series of experiments on dogs. They kept one group of dogs awake for days on end, tying their collars to a wall so that the animals could not lie down. Then they killed the dogs and extracted fluid from their spinal canals, believing this fluid to be rich in 'hypnotoxins' — an endogenous sleep-inducing chemical that had built up inside the dogs' bodies over the days and nights of prolonged wakefulness. Legendre and Piéron injected this fluid into healthy dogs and found that without exception the dogs swiftly fell asleep. Their hunch so easily confirmed, they rushed to announce that they had stumbled upon, or so they believed, their very own sleep potion.

I would like to know if hypnotoxins are real. Or if they ought to be classed alongside phlogiston and aether, or any number of other material causes fantasised into existence by science. Then again, perhaps hypnotoxins belong elsewhere entirely, with the ontological inventions of Perrault, Andersen, and Grimm.

Another student of sleep swayed by the idea of hypnotoxins was Constantin von Economo, the Romanian-born medical doctor who named the mysterious sleeping sickness that broke out in 1917 and, over the course of the next decade, caused the deaths of some five million people across the globe. The pandemic sounds like something a Bond villain might concoct, or like a novel by José Saramago, in that suddenly people began suffering raging fevers and experiencing hallucinations, before falling into spells of prolonged sleep from which it was near-impossible to rouse them. Many of them subsequently died (mostly in their sleep, but occasionally in states of sleeplessness so acute as to preclude sedation). This was a wicked enchantment indeed.

Von Economo's sickness, *encephalitis lethargica*, became the subject of Oliver Sacks's *Awakenings*, a deeply affecting clinical work that grew out of Sacks's treatment, in 1969, of a number of the original surviving patients, plunged into a real-life equivalent of enchanted sleep. Unresponsive, immobile, speechless, closed off from and indifferent to the world around them, these patients were awakened, as if by magic, by the administering of levodopa. Coming to life after more than forty years, like fairy-tale characters clicked out of suspended animation by a kiss, they reinhabited their identities as if nothing had happened, as if whole decades had not passed them by. They were astute, engaged, communicative, full of hopes and plans, and then, one by one, when the effects of levodopa proved temporary, they fell back into an inert state, under the somnolent spell of their sickness.

One patient, Leonard L., tried to cram as much life as he'd been swindled out of into his temporary 'awakening'. He chased down sensation in all its forms, soaked up every savour. Sacks notes, 'Everything about him filled him with delight: he was like a man who had awoken from a nightmare or a serious illness, or a man released from entombment or prison, who is suddenly intoxicated with the sense and beauty of everything around him.' Leonard L. was drunk on reality. Going out into the hospital gardens, he would touch the flowers and leaves and bend to kiss them. He began to take taxi rides through New York City by night, each time returning breathless with excitement over the neon-doused sights. When he read Dante's *Paradiso*, it was with tears of joy in his eyes. 'I feel saved,' he told Sacks, 'resurrected, re-born. I feel a sense of health amounting to Grace . . . I feel like a man in love.'

It didn't last. Sacks recounts how this excess of living, this '*too-muchness*', soon overwhelmed Leonard L. It tipped him over the edge. The grace turned to mania, thence to messianic delusion. After forty years spent sleeping, this is understandable.

I am genuinely moved by Leonard L.'s mania and self-inflation, by a surpassing *joie de vivre* that is admirable, if not in fact enviable. Who, after all, hasn't hankered after a little too-muchness? It is his crashing, domino-like cascade into diminishment that floors me. First his inner and outer thoughts became increasingly libidinal. Leonard L. would wake hollering from erotic dreams, while by day his yearnings tormented him. He was full of lewd talk, groped the nurses, and masturbated freely. He developed a number of tics, initially around the eyes, but soon there appeared 'grimaces, cluckings and lightning-quick scratchings'. He grew overly familiar and overly loquacious, then urgent, compulsive, obsessional. Six weeks into his treatment, Leonard L. wrote a 50,000-word autobiography — 'typing ceaselessly', high as a kite. Yet within a month Sacks found him in state of suicidal depression, besieged by thoughts of torture, death, and castration. When suddenly it all came to a stop Leonard L. reverted to his original motionless state. Thereafter he scarcely spoke.

Later, during a rare moment when he was able to summon words, Leonard L. told Sacks that levodopa was
the devil's drug. Given the choice he would side with
the dark.

When von Economo dissected the brains of people who
had perished from sleeping sickness back in the 1920s
he found that most of them exhibited damage in the
hypothalamus region of the brain. He conjectured that
the hypothalamus acted as a kind of neural sleep-control
centre. Then as now, if you stimulate the hypothalamus
you can make people fall asleep.

If sleep science could probe the brain of Sleeping
Beauty — surely a sleeping sickness victim before the fact,
snoozing for a hundred years, dead to the world — what
might it find? Would her hypothalamus be enlarged, the
result of being forced into endocrine overdrive? And what
sort of brain-wave function would Beauty display when
hooked up to electrodes? On the hunt for some mysterious 'sleep substance' or sleep-inducing hypnotoxin, our
imaginary sleep scientists might detect culpable levels of
adenosine or serotonin, or growth-hormone-releasing
hormone — all shown to cause drowsiness — to say nothing of that pop-medical panacea, melatonin.

But perhaps I am running ahead of myself, given that the organ that was sleeping in the fair princess was not her brain but her heart.

Buscot Park, in Oxfordshire, lies eighty-five miles north-west of London. Dominated by a handsome grey-stone manor house set on a rise amid sweeping Italianate gardens, the estate, belonging to Lord Faringdon, is now partly in the care of the National Trust. Here, in an eclectic saloon too ornate for my tastes (Empire furniture, Murano chandelier, gilt-edged wall panels), hangs a series of four monumental paintings that narrate the story of 'Little Briar Rose'. They are the work — arguably the life work, since their subject preoccupied him for close on forty years — of the Late Pre-Raphaelite painter Edward Burne-Jones. When first exhibited in London, in 1890, at Agnew & Sons in Bond Street then at Toynbee Hall, the paintings caused a sensation. Visitors mesmerised by their luminous colour, rich with forest greens, royal reds, and lapis blue, fell to gasping. Spellbound by seductive compositional lines that arc across the panels in languorous arabesques and lead the eye on through twisting briars and the folding drapes of the council room arras to the curtained bower where the princess slumbers, they swooned. The actress Ellen Terry was, for her part, reduced to tears.

Another visitor, claiming to have been 'transported' by the paintings, reported that he would never forget the crowds of 'well-dressed women' who sat in silence in front of the panels, 'so immoveable that it would have been easy to fancy that they had all been pricked by the fatal fairy spindle, and were all sleeping beauties themselves'.

Ah, that fatal spindle. I know it well. It has lived in my memories of childhood for as long as I can remember. My father was a couturier (which qualifies him as a wizard of sorts, a magician of appearances), and although there were no fairy spindles at home on which to prick my finger, there were plenty of pins lying around, buried in the weave of the carpet, left over from endless evenings spent hemming and tucking. An innocent hazard, you might think, for a child running around barefoot. Yet each time I stepped on a pin, and there were many times, I feared setting loose some malicious spirit as I watched, transfixed, the tiny red sphere of virgin blood ooze from my pricked heel.

What if I told you that I came to Buscot Park to dispel just that sort of dream, one that clouds my vision and makes it gauzy, overlaying my actual feelings about Briar Rose with afterthoughts as obscuring as cataracts?

Nudged on by insomnia, I had somehow persuaded myself that beauty in repose represents something aspirational — a barely attainable ideal maybe, or quality of perfection, I don't know. But, here, now, I had no intention of being transported out of place and time to some frozen fairy-tale limbo, like those well-dressed Victorian women who swooned. I wanted to wake myself up. Standing before Burne-Jones's handmaidens dozing beside the well, or slumped asleep over the idle loom (whose 'restless shuttle lieth still'), I fought the paintings' supine allure. And I failed entirely to connect to the passive princess, transfigured by sleep, no longer a person but a gift — or conduit, or key, something, at any rate, transactional.

Glad to be jogged out of my revisionist reveries, I remembered that the princess who had captured my heart as a child was insomniac — utterly incapable of sleeping even when perched atop of tower of mattresses. Her restlessness was ostensibly the outward manifestation of her possessing a sensibility so refined that she could feel a single pea trapped beneath the bottom mattress.

But I knew better. I knew that this princess was just another ordinary, bad-tempered little girl. In my experience, it is generous-minded but not uncommon to see refinement where in fact there is only neurosis.

Besides, real sleep is not perfect in its stillness. Bodies are not impeccable in repose. If you were to secure a camera to the ceiling above your bed and let it roll, the following day you would be able to treat yourself to a night-time's choreography of rolling and unrolling, flipping, grunting, coughing, jerking, kicking, snoring, snorting, masturbating, and dreaming. In sleep we are neither beautiful nor restful.

A vein of memory opened up at Buscot Park, of tantrums and sulks, connivings and deceits, for I could not abide sleep when I was small. Genuinely terrified of the blank negation it imposed, I would exert myself to come up with fresh ways to dodge the bedtime curfew — every evening a different excuse. At lights-out, a minor rebellion. At six, I knew that sleep was a cursed thing sent to bring the curtain down on the material pleasures of my world — on play, adventuring, company, and the fizzing, bubble-forming activity of thought itself. It was my nemesis (as surely as torchlight was a friend). Squirming in my narrow bed, consumed with fiery refusal, I determined that I would not submit myself to sleep — or, as I saw it then, to disappearing. If sleep wanted to claim me, it would jolly well have to snatch me.

When Burne-Jones painted his Briar Rose cycle, grown women who had too much to say and to do were being forcibly put to bed. They were diagnosed as hysterics, depressives and neurasthenics, whose delicate nerves were no match for their mental gymnastics, and given a prescription of hardcore rest. Many of these women were insomniac. Some had eating disorders, others were suicidal. To a woman (almost) they balked at the societal restrictions that corralled them into being mothers and homemakers and disallowed anything else. Nervous conditions, sleeplessness, self-starvation (that is, disappearing before you are made to disappear), this was their protest.

Another epiphany. As a child I understood very well that Beauty's cursed sleep was wrought by ugliness's jealousy. By ugliness being excluded from the charmed circle. At the time I could not have known why I found this so troubling. But life without ugly is a flat and monotone thing not worth having. It is every bit as vapid as enchanted sleep.

Zzz and I have lately been facing down a good deal of ugly. Friends dying unexpectedly and before their time, elderly relatives stricken and compromised by age and illness, the ructions and traumas of family upheavals that have forced upon us an elasticity we didn't know we possessed. It has brought us closer. Taught us how pointless it is to set up defences against the pain of just living.

For better and for worse, for richer and for poorer. These are the matrimonial vows that Zzz and I never wanted to make — another version of accepting both the beautiful and the ugly. We thought it was enough to make a marriage bed and to root ourselves in it.

There was, as you would expect, an actual physical bed, the one Zzz bought to welcome me over the threshold of his solitariness. Proudly, he told me that it came with a Sealy mattress, which alone had set him back six hundred dollars (a princely sum all those years ago). The bed ate up half the available floor space in the tiny one-room studio that Zzz had rented in Palo Alto, after moving on from a marriage that had failed to thrive. I slept soundly in that bed, but Zzz did not. Until then we had conducted our relationship in episodic bursts, enjoying intense but circumscribed weeks of connection, with one or the other of us flying across the Atlantic every few months to dive into the other's world. Now, along with a large shipment of books and paintings, two suitcases full of clothing, and sundry other belongings — my trusty clock, a beat-up (I thought of it as 'seasoned') coffee machine, a few favourite throws — that I had uprooted so as to make myself feel more at home, I was there to stay. The order of things had been overturned and Zzz wasn't entirely sure the new configuration suited him.

What do I remember about those early weeks in Palo Alto? Not much, if truth be told, since within a month we had moved again, into a roomier apartment in San Francisco. I remember how funny I thought it was that as you came into the small downtown area, jammed with restaurants catering to Palo Alto's affluent populace, you would be enveloped by an aromatic cloud of warm vented air, mellow with garlic and herbs. And I remember walking those same streets when Zzz was at work, feeling lonelier than I had ever felt. I would dip in and out of boutique shops, craftsy and overpriced, most of them, and make small talk with the staff, trying on a transatlantic twang and experimenting with the idea of belonging.

A better, more visceral memory is of sliding into a red-leatherette-lined booth at the old-fashioned creamery — Zzz opposite me, smiling, spoon at the ready. The place offered twin thrills, both time travel and fakery. The plastic seat covering stuck to my thighs, my skin peeling off it with a squeak, and the waitresses wore updos from which coy ringlets tumbled, and white frilled aprons, like they'd stepped out of a 1950s sitcom. Zzz would order the knickerbocker glory, or at least its American equivalent, an ice-cream boat of such grandiose proportions it would arrive laden with multiple scoops of dairy ice, whole bananas, crenellated whipped-cream caterpillars that ran all over the show, and a confetti throw of sprinkles and popping candy. Diving in with my spoon to work one end of the confection as Zzz worked the other, I ate like a champ. I ate for England.

Palto Alto boasts a famous Art Deco movie palace, saved from closure by one of the founders of Hewlett-Packard (I forget which), and it really, truly had a man rising up from the pit beneath the screen playing a Wurlitzer organ to the accompaniment of flashing lights, and grinning madly over his shoulder as he scanned the open-mouthed faces of the bewildered audience behind him. It was like the bizarre wedding serenade Zzz and I never had.

Twenty years on, as part of a bid to wake up to each other anew, Zzz and I have adopted a new bedroom — a home from home in the Balearic Islands. It is part of a (badly) converted grain store that sits above the original olive press belonging to a centuries-old rural *finca*, and it is full of heavy dark-wood furniture. There is a linen chest worthy of a bridal trousseau and a weighty bed that looks as though it ought to be curtained, instead of lying bare under the solid wood beams that hold up the ceiling. This is a bedroom for all seasons. However, it is especially resonant when our upstairs neighbour uses her sink, because whenever she does so it rains in the closet. The first time this happened Zzz's mono hearing sounded a panicked alarm. But once we caught on to the anomaly, we began to open the cupboard door whenever it 'rained' then climb back into bed to view the spectacle. The indoor rain was a pitter-patter metaphor for containing the pain of just living.

The writer Charlotte Perkins Gilman described how at Silas Weir Mitchell's Philadelphia clinic, in the spring of 1887, she was 'put to bed and kept there'. Mitchell was the physician who devised the infamous rest cure, after working with soldiers who had emerged from the Civil War afflicted with 'wounded nerves'. When he later applied his treatment to women who complained of nervous disorders, he embellished his strict regimen of bed rest, combining it with massage, electrotherapy, and fat-filled diets. During the first ten days undergoing his cure, Mitchell insisted that his women patients were fed on milk alone, like babies.

This is Mitchell itemising the cardinal points of the rest cure: 'I do not permit the patient to sit up, or to sew or write or read, or to use the hands in any active way except to clean the teeth . . . I arrange to have the bowels and water passed while lying down, and the patient is lifted on to a lounger for an hour in the morning and again at bedtime, and then lifted back again into the newly-made bed.' And this is Perkins Gilman writing in her diary on the eve of her admission to Mitchell's clinic: 'I am very sick with nervous prostration, and I think with some brain disease as well. No one can ever know what I have suffered in these last five years. Pain pain pain, till my mind has given way.' The difference in his use of language and hers is heart-stopping. It bespeaks of worlds violently colliding.

As you might guess, the rest cure did little to relieve Charlotte's suffering, save remove her temporarily from an unhappy marriage and the nagging feeling of having failed as a mother. It gave her a safe space, which even she briefly acknowledged to be a respite. Rest was no bad thing, she conceded, if it served as a spur to further activity.

But no sooner was Charlotte discharged and sent home than her symptoms redoubled. Years later she would write in her autobiography that the rest cure had caused her almost to lose her mind. She didn't. But for purposes of what she termed 'pure propaganda' (and of a distinctly feminist flavor), she decided that the neurasthenic woman at the centre of her short story 'The Yellow Wallpaper' should lose hers.

Gilman's unnamed fictional heroine undergoes a harrowing rest cure of her own, in which she is beset by florid hallucinations that play across the hideous wallpaper — all 'bulbous eyes' and suicidal swirls: 'like a broken neck' — of the attic room where she has been put to bed. As these swirling shapes coalesce in her mind she sees patterns slowly emerge, of bars, and then behind these bars she spies a ghostly woman creeping, stopping every so often to shake her cage. Unable to free herself, the phantasm keeps on with her creeping until eventually the rest-cure patient joins her. Having scratched off most of the wallpaper, she falls to crawling round and round the room, seeking escape. She is on her knees. The rest cure has brought her low.

In his will William Shakespeare left his wife, Anne Hathaway, his 'second best bed'. We don't know for sure who got the best one (possibly his daughter Susanna). Nor do we know much about the bedrock of Shakespeare's marriage.

Feminist scholars squabble over the meaning of this bequest. There are those who feel chagrined on Anne's behalf and insist that the second-best bed he left to his wife implies his second-rate regard. They may be right, since historically the marriage bed was the most important of chattels, and often it was the most valuable item of furniture a couple owned. Then again, perhaps these scholars are just bogged down by literalism.

The marriage bed represents infinite trust. This is something Penelope grasped at her very core. It is why, when crushed by doubt, suspicious that the man returned to Ithaca after twenty years (cunningly disguised) might not after all be her husband, she decides to test him. She orders her maidservant to pull Odysseus's bed onto the terrace, the better to make him comfortable for the night, even as she knows that the bed cannot be moved because it has been partially carved from a living olive tree (by Odysseus himself) that is rooted in the very foundations of the house. Still, she makes sure he is within earshot as she issues her command. She wants him to feel his jeopardy, to understand that moving the bed would entail killing the tree and, by implication, their marriage. Moving the bed would bring their house down!

Instantly the power dynamic between the couple is reversed, for while Penelope's hesitation over Odysseus's identity might belie her lack of faith, this business with the bed effectively transfers the burden of proof to his shoulders. It is no longer Penelope's loyalty that is on trial (judged by whether or not she knows him), but his own (tested by whether or not, having well and truly strayed, he knows his marriage bed when he sees it).

In the eyes of some classical scholars, this trial by bed only ramps up the case for Penelope's wiliness. But Penelope's mind is confused — 'She wept for her own husband, who was right next to her', as Emily Wilson's new translation of *The Odyssey* has it. And since she cannot think, she acts. The way I see it, the possibility that Penelope might finally have been granted the very thing she has longed for nonstop, for two whole decades, is so overwhelming that misgivings surge through her like a stress hormone, overriding hope.

The poet Stephen Cushman finds the shifting meanings of the marriage bed to be equally potent — and perhaps, equally confusing. 'Behold the wreckage of night,' he writes, inviting us to picture 'covers disheveled by love'. Or if not love, then anxiety, in which case the bedclothes may have been cast off 'in vast deserts of insomnia where trepidations bomb tranquility to rubble'. Cushman does not elaborate. But in observing how the bed — this 'hub of marriage' — got mangled, he advises that we remake it, and that we bring care and deliberation to the task. He suggests we think about solemnising the occasion, working to God's plan or 'Noah's pattern' and bringing in male and female, two by two, to ensure renewal.

In Cushman's view, the marriage bed is an ark in its own right — a divinely blessed covenant that consecrates coupledom. By remaking it we can remake the world. And night will be its witness.

At Buscot Park it was Burne-Jones's handsome prince who persistently drew my gaze — the only wakeful figure in all the paintings. Poised at the far end of the first panel, a knight clad in iron plating, he stands with his sword at the ready, surveying the thorny briar in whose tangled branches are suspended the twisted bodies of those who went before him only to perish, and contemplates how he is going to 'smite the sleeping world awake'. I would like you please to note that the prince does not wish to kiss or smooch the world awake. He wants to make a noise and shake it the hell up, like Gilgamesh.

Or like Burne-Jones himself. Or like his political compadre, William Morris. The former, so often dismissed as a dreamer or idealist who longed to escape the world into a mythic past of fairy tales and Arthurian lore, in reality nurtured the dearly held hope of creating a contemporary revolution in art and vision. Morris, meanwhile (and it was Morris who penned the verses I've been quoting, mourning the stillness of the 'restless shuttle' and calling on the prince to smite the world awake), threw in his lot with the exploited proletariat. Both men recognised that enchanted sleep is dreamless. And if you can't dream, then how can you entertain visions of a better world? *How can you incite revolutions?*

In my CBT group there were about fifteen insomniacs with assorted complaints. A man with the lofty but stooped bearing of a Romantic poet, pale and bony-faced and so wired he could not sleep at all. A woman who kept falling asleep at her office desk, but stayed up all night watching Netflix. Another woman whose issues remained murky: red-eyed, hunted-looking, she would cry each time she was invited to share something personal. Perhaps we were all thwarted revolutionaries, exhausted by the fight, as battle-weary as Gilgamesh but without the euphoric kick. I mean, the energy in that room was as flat as days-old beer.

If only Charles Simic had been there to share the joke. Here, at last, I had stumbled upon his congress of insomniacs. We were not a glamorous bunch. Gathered in a hospital conference room, not a ballroom, and with no starry speakers about to take the stage, we had to content ourselves with padded blue institutional chairs, wide-beamed and pilling, sugary drinks, and cheap biscuits — the kind of surroundings that can build a tentative camaraderie based on head-shaking incredulity. Here were the zombies: and here was the nice room where we would sit in a circle and try not to growl.

At the sleep clinic we learned about sleep and how to get it. We learned to keep sleep diaries and we learned about sleep hygiene. All of us were given sleep diets.

I told the group that I had been reading Samuel Pepys's diary, which recorded his nocturnal escapades, modest as they were in being confined to his bedchamber. Still, Pepys relates how all the world came to him. His bed was a place for music and reading, and when he deigned to share it with guests who had come to dine and then overstayed, it was where their diverting conversation continued. Pepys liked to get his hair cut in his bedchamber by a trusted female servant (who had to put up with the occasional grope), and he routinely quarrelled and reconciled with his wife beneath the covers. When things were good between them he would teach Mrs Pepys 'things in astronomy' under a gibbous moon, vigilant as a peeled eyeball.

Pepys's busy bedchamber went against every tenet of sleep hygiene, whose humourless adherents insist that beds are for two things alone, sleep and sex.

Going by the rules of sleep hygiene, Zzz and I make for wholly incompatible bedfellows. I like to leave the window open for ventilation; he likes it shut (else every footfall on pavement, bird call, or car alarm gets funnelled into his one hearing ear). I long for an immersive darkness, he leaves the bedroom door open to bothersome light from the stairwell, claiming this generates the airflow that I would much rather blew in from outside. I feel the cold; he gets hot and bothered. He reads past midnight, I pass out with my book falling on my face, and when I snore he elbows me. However, going by the more forgiving rules of love, Zzz and I accommodate each other, in sleep as in life.

The modern cure for insomnia is sleep restriction. The opposite of the rest cure, which feeds you up, the sleep diet keeps you hungry for sleep by keeping things lean. How lean, you might ask? Well, first you need to work out how much sleep you are entitled to by determining your 'sleep-efficiency quotient' — a magic number arrived at by dividing the number of hours you sleep by the number of hours you actually spend in bed, trying and failing to sleep. My sleep quotient is 63 per cent, so my diet is strict. It obliges me to sleep for no more than the 5.6 hours a night that I averaged over a four-week run, diligently recorded in the sleep diary I'd been encouraged to keep at the sleep clinic. Only if I up my sleep-efficiency quotient to 90 per cent by observing proper sleep-hygiene practices am I permitted to add fifteen minutes of sleep to my nightly diet.

It is a torment to take an insomniac and then deprive them of sleep. The sleep therapists seem entirely blind to the fact that counting anything, but most of all counting sleep — calculating its efficiency, its depth, its span, while adding up every minute spent lying awake each night between all-too-shallow bouts of it — is the very thing that will stop an insomniac from sleeping. That, or they are sadists.

Nor do the sleep experts, who freely advise on cognitive matters (the C in CBT), appreciate the workings of the insomniac mind. Routinely, they offer the sleep-deprived a range of 'blockers' to counter those insistent, intrusive thoughts that can keep us from sleeping. One of these blockers consists of silently chanting 'the, the, the, the, the', over and over, for unendurably long minutes. It is the mental equivalent of telling your brain to talk to the hand. And yet 'the, the, the, the, the' is just the sort of senseless thought-train that nourishes the insomniac mind: repetitive, rhythmic, dumbly enigmatic and therefore intrinsically engaging, it pivots between the familiar and alien, zooms in and out of the uncanny.

Besides, intrusive thinking is just one way the insomniac brain stokes itself. Harder to fathom (and to treat) is the freewheeling, seemingly autonomous tripping through utter banality, the night-time regurgitation of daytime crud — of the stuff that doesn't actually merit deliberation — that moves like an arm-linked chain of can-can dancers through a demi-wakefulness that exists beyond any conscious control, but (and this is the source of frustration) is conscious enough — kick, and kick, and kick — that you have to clock it.

Too often my insomniac mind is stuck in crud-chewing mode. It feeds me snippets of song, meshed with advertorial-type sloganising that might, in turn, trigger a memory from childhood before pinging back to a thought-of desire (a want) or to something I saw on the internet, or something someone told me — then on again, unpredictable, inconsequential, threading and worming inside my head. Nothing is more inimical to rest and yet I am powerless to stop it. It is like waterboarding the mind with meaningless overflow, a smothering drip, drip, drip of surplus thought.

It is a well-known fact that each of us contains an internal clock that regulates our circadian rhythms (in response to changing levels of temperature, light, and melatonin, among other things). These cellular clocks have just two modes, wakeful and sleepy, roughly corresponding to day and night, but in insomniacs they don't work properly, the likely result of irregularities in melatonin production. When your circadian rhythms are out of sync with the diurnal round, you feel sleepy at odd, inconvenient times and awake at night: jet-lagged in your native time zone. Strictly speaking, these body clocks are not a timekeeping device but a sleepkeeping one, a guardian of the rest that each of us is permitted to accrue.

When I think of insomnia's wayward rhythms what I picture is this: gaudy insomnia with its wide lapels and toothy grin is the last groover on the dance floor, still going at it after everyone else has collapsed in a heap or gone home. You are desperate to shut up the joint for the night but insomnia is on a roll, singing along to all the tunes, gyrating wildly, body popping and whooping, letting it rip. To crown it all, insomnia is a god-awful dancer. You are wilting with exhaustion. Bleary-eyed, your body leaden, you hanker for nothing more than to sleep, and yet you must endure this thing — this coked-up arriviste! — who on top of everything else (the clowning, the nagging insistence, the manic glare) has no freaking beats.

Neither do I, as it happens. In menopause I have grown accustomed to having no rhythms to speak of, neither hormonal nor lunar, and certainly not circadian.

Still, there are other rhythms that govern sleep, subject to such complex mechanisms of internal control that the best we can do is represent them graphically. I am referring to those characteristic patterns of electrical activity that the brain displays as it stealthily guides us into sleep, beta waves morphing into alpha waves then theta waves, and finally delta waves — those long-drawn-out pulses that scratch extended claw marks onto the graph paper and signify the arrival of deep sleep. Reading up on this process, a joyful thump pulses my chest as I learn that at the threshold of sleep, on the very brink of delta-wave insensibility, you get a blip or two on the graph, which on closer inspection turns out to be a series of shallow theta waves, all bunched up like yarn wound around a spindle. Without these 'sleep spindles' forming, sleep will not come. So perhaps every sleep is enchanted after all.

Except for REM sleep. Which is not enchanted but paradoxical, because in REM sleep the body sleeps deeply while the brain is only half-sleeping. This explains why we can snap out of a bad dream, or spring awake in the middle of a too-good one, and why, once in a rare blue moon, we experience the strange power trip that is lucid dreaming. The paradoxes inherent in REM sleep, however, cannot even begin to account for how the brain is able to entertain itself with its own magic-lantern shows, raiding the image banks of our unconscious minds, searching out characters and props and wholly repressed memories and motivations, and then knit them together into spontaneously evolving storylines and dissolving phantasmagoria.

In October 1964, Vladimir Nabokov decided to keep a dream diary. Every morning, immediately upon waking, he would write down whatever he could rescue from the night, and for the next couple of days he would be on active lookout for anything that seemed to do with the remembered dream. Nabokov was testing a theory which suggested that dreams might be prophetic; that rather than containing a jumble of reconstituted shards of daily experience, mingled with cut-and-paste plots borrowed from our memory stores and personal demons escaped from the inner closets of repression, our dreams might also offer a proleptic vision of what is to come, turning every one of us into clairvoyants.

Nabokov had fallen under the sway of the maverick British aeronautical engineer John W. Dunne, who, in the early decades of the last century, came up with a left-field theory of Time that he laid out in a series of cryptic books filled with runic runs of algebra and frenetic diagrams. Boiled down to its concentrate by one Nabokov scholar, the theory posits that 'time's progress is not unidirectional but recursive: the reason we do not notice the backflow is that we are not paying attention'. In 1964, Nabokov started paying attention, and he recorded several instances of *identifying preamnesia* — that is, unwittingly manufacturing a preceding dream that matched a later waking experience. For Nabokov, as for Dunne, dreams became a kind of portal through which chunks of personal experience could effectively be teleported across time.

In this topsy-turvy world in which time can multiply serially or run backwards inside hidden loops, dreams are to timekeeping what wormholes are to space. They are singularities into which all succession (with wormholes, its dimension) simply pours and is obliterated. The question is whether insomnia might also qualify as a singularity, and, if so, what gets sucked in and obliterated other than sleep. Peace of mind, rest, a coherent sense of one's self? Or is it your dignity?

Roberto Bolaño wrote of the numberless ways in which those shapeless border zones between one place and another (Texas and Mexico, in his case, but it could be anywhere, and it could be day and night) mess with your head. The borderlands are neither here nor there, neither this nor that. They are a no-man's-land patrolled by vigilantes and assassins. The soil under your feet in the borderlands is watered with blood and the horizons offer only 'wind and dust' — a 'minimal dream'. Such places (or psychic spaces), says Bolaño, lead to a condition that is much to be feared. He calls it an 'eviction of the mind'.

Another dream theory: our dreams are social. Which is to say there exist dream templates we all share, born of mythic archetypes that reside in the collective un-

conscious (thank you, Jung) or arising out of shared
traumatic experiences of the kind that Charlotte Beradt
uncovered in the 1930s, when as a young Jewish journalist living in Vienna she suffered nightmares of being
'hunted from pillar to post — shot at, tortured, scalped'.
Convinced that her countrymen and women were, like
her, busy funnelling their anxieties into their dreams, she
began to interview people about their nightmares and
to write these down. Synergies and sympathies quickly
emerged, leading Beradt to conclude that people who
live in fear for their freedom under stridently authori-
tarian regimes end up inhabiting a shared dreamscape.
'In the darkness of night they reproduced in distortion
all they had experienced in that sinister daytime world.'

One woman dreamt that posters had been set up on
every street corner listing the words people were no
longer permitted to use. The first was *Lord*, the last, *I*.
Neither god nor self could be acknowledged. Another
person dreamt he was in his apartment relaxing with a
book, when suddenly the walls around his room then
his apartment disappear, and he hears over a loud-
speaker that henceforth the Nazis are outlawing all
walls. He told Beradt: 'I looked around and discovered
to my horror that as far as the eye could see, no apartment had walls anymore.' Beradt claims that this is

the dream of someone who resists collectivisation. It is rooted in a defiance that would lead to a sanity-saving dissociation: what people at the time began to call 'Inner Emigration'.

In many of the dreams — Beradt smuggled them out of Austria after the *Anschluss* of 1938, scrawled in code on tiny bits of paper — the domestic space that ought to safeguard an individual's privacy becomes a place of terror and surveillance. Lamps listen to you then tell you off, cushions balk, spying desk clocks testify against you. One of Beradt's subjects dreamt that the Dutch oven in her living room 'began to talk in a harsh and penetrating voice, repeating every word she and her husband said against the government'.

Coping with the mounting paranoia (a symptomatic shunting of the logic of insomnia into day) demanded urgent measures. Not so much an inner emigration but its opposite, an inner evacuation. This could take a sinister turn, making people blind — asleep! — to the atrocities being enacted all around them. Elsewise, it might befuddle and confound the authorities, as one woman envisioned when she dreamt that she was talking in her sleep and 'to be on the safe side' was talking in Russian — a language she neither spoke nor understood. If she could not understand herself, she reasoned, then neither could the government. Unconsciously, the woman sought subterfuge from the fascists by making herself unintelligible. This is also an eviction of the mind.

In a coda to the English translation of Beradt's dream collection, published in 1966, Bruno Bettelheim observes that the Nazi regime successfully forced its enemies to dream the kind of dreams it wanted them to dream. That resistance was impossible, that they were contaminated and inferior, that safety lay only in compliance. These were dreams that told people too much about themselves. They were dreams that told them what they did not want to know. On this account, writes Bettelheim, the Nazis, like Macbeth, 'murdered sleep'.

I could murder some sleep. Even at the price of reckoning with my soul. Especially at that price, in fact, since everybody carries a part of the night within them, a small piece of impenetrable, unknowing darkness, akin to what Freud referred to as the 'navel' of a dream, which was his term for that untranslatable nub of the thing that forever resists interpretation.

The other night I had a shotgun awakening, courtesy of a bad dream that refused to end and instead seeped out of my head and into the bedroom like a noxious gas, contaminating everything. Whatever I peered at in the dark acquired jagged edges or some other menacing aspect: furniture loomed, taking on fearsome dimensions. The curtains looked shifty. Even Zzz looked unnaturally angular in shadowy outline, as though some nocturnal Medusa had slunk her snaky head around our bedroom door and ossified him mid-rollover. Never had Zzz's absence appeared more present. Looking at him — looking for him — was like looking into the abyss.

It is at moments like these, when I sense the void migrate from the perimeter of my existence and begin to pervade its centre, that I start to question what I am about. Why am I in this house, this bed, this marriage? Why, when I look back over a string of formative selves, all those era-defined embodiments of me pulling in different directions, do I find myself on this path and not on any other? What time-bending tricks has life played on me? I have honoured every emotional contract I was signatory to and yet I seem to have lost myself. At moments such as these, everything that is closest to my heart, that generates the impression of gravity in my world, gets rudely pitched across the universe.

Unable to calm myself, I tiptoe down to the basement kitchen to bide my time with the dog. In the bone-white light of almost-dawn we snuggle up together on the sofa, fur against skin, warming each other up, and he huffs his satisfaction, indistinguishable from an old man's sigh. It sounds delusional, but in those night-waking hours spent with the dog I am convinced that he understands me. Perhaps he intuits that because I spend all my days transmitting, at night I wish only to receive.

This being the case, I wonder if it is even possible for messages to communicate themselves across the void. Can the universe thrum its reassurances over a distance from which everything molecular, everything that has substance and mass and meaning, has been expelled? I wish I knew.

This morning the dog kept his distance and I can't say that I blame him. Bloodless and inert (more vampire than zombie), and drained of wants, I sat at the table coddling a mug of lukewarm coffee. As I felt myself shrink from London's thin grey light, it occurred to me that were I to fix myself to the spot as the sun gradually burned through the cloud cover to focus its bright rays on the panes in my kitchen window, I might well fizzle into an inky puddle of smoking dung, too sour even to be of use to the garden.

The nightmare that woke me was like all the others, authored by anxiety, barely worth recalling. In every one of this species of angst-driven dream I am variously thwarted: handicapped, delayed, misread, felled by illness, accident, or violence. I am endlessly diverted and distracted, trapped in a mirrored hall. Every time it is the same. Happenstance foils me, my voice gets scrambled or I am thrown obstacles I cannot surmount. These dreams never fail to trip my pulse and make me breathe hard and shallow. Frequently they are more exhausting than the missed sleep that arrives in their wake.

By my own diagnosis, my neurotic tendencies have run amok across my dreamscape, infusing tension and upset into the simplest chain of events, breaking the chain, disrupting the flow of causality, frustrating intent. My dream-space is an untrustworthy place. At any moment it might fold up on itself along invisible fissures, like speeded-up origami, creating new and disturbing portals and vistas. Or else it dissolves away in front of me, holes flowering open onto darkness the way acid corrodes cinematic tape. My dreams show up the seams of my reality, and sometimes they split open its skin like a burst fruit.

I know that in our dreams night and day are in conversation, arguing point and counterpoint, hammering out the problems of existence. But still.

At least our dreams are social. At least our neuroses are shared. I take some comfort knowing this. I also take comfort from the knowledge that our most important dreams and perhaps, especially, nightmares tend to recur, for as Gertrude Stein famously said: 'there is no such thing as repetition, only insistence'. Sometimes the unconscious just has to be heard.

A shrink I know once told me matter-of-factly that people tend to fall in love with their neuroses. *That must be why they come to see you*, I remember telling him at the time: *they want to be cured of this wayward love*. But now I think that being in love with our neuroses is what makes us human. It lends us our individuality and distinctiveness, our particular angles, edges, and quirks.

Because I am able to look at my own insomnia (not objectively — who can do that when it comes to so subversive an experience? — but critically) I recognise it to be the product of excess. An excess of longing and an excess of thinking. Of course, my insomnia is to a large extent also a First World, post-capitalist artefact, although knowing this is of little use to me. What does help, what does ease the overdrive, is when I try to leach insomnia's power over me by siphoning off my looping night-time thoughts and straightening them out into ordered words on the page, *physicalising* them. I get up, in other words, and I write.

But then the fear that presses in on me is that my work might be fated never to transcend the neurotic. The very idea that this may be the case is so profoundly disturbing, so unsettling, it is as if the ground I walk on had begun to bubble and liquefy. Writing for me is both compass and anchor.

Writing is also one of the few observances — sleep being an obvious other — that gets me beyond myself. Gets me 'out of the way', as we say in creative writing classes. Some people meditate, I write.

However, if my writing is ultimately neurotic then when I finally do rediscover the art of sleeping will the wellspring of my creativity run dry?

This is where a taxonomy of darkness comes to the rescue. It starts by acknowledging all the strange things that can be seen and felt in insomnia, not just its frights and distortions but its visions and intimations — the frayed thread-ends of one's own existence, to instance one of its ambivalent gifts. Or, just sometimes, just maybe, the faintly detectable buzz of a cosmic hum that was there before human beings came into existence and will be there until the end of time.

How can I characterise those frayed thread-ends for you? (Where not even the Fates could find enough to work with in spinning the future.)

It is tricky. As soon as you reach for them, they retract. However, in glancing fashion they reveal themselves along the fringe-tips of your perception or they encroach stealthwise upon your bodily extremities like a sudden chill. In such moments you sense with absolute clarity exactly where the reliable plotlines of your life terminate. You are dangling over the precipice and it feels like falling.

Or you become supremely aware of the particular way that your exposed head, poking out from under the duvet, confronts the uncertain night air. Your breath escapes in warm puffs into a nothingness you cannot apprehend and that offers nothing in the way of resistance; and yet a proprioceptive sense of precisely where your head is located in space, all the pressure points acting on it, where it weighs heavy on the pillow, where it brushes against the edge of the sheet, is so painfully acute it is as if your entire being had taken up residence in your cranium. All of you imbues a singular Nowness that has amplitude and mass, and nothing else exists.

Approached another way, the sense of precarity I am trying to convey might manifest itself as a feeling of otherness in the ankles or the underside of your feet, arising at those times when you are lying awake unable to find any tolerable posture of repose. Your extremities become hypersensitised, agitated, but also lumpen and foreign. Rationally you comprehend that these outlying appendages belong to you, are part of you. But at the same time you are exquisitely aware that they somehow need reclaiming from the night.

We are strangers to nocturnality much of the time, and not merely because we absent ourselves from night. We want to believe that natural magic and not the permissiveness of darkness strings spider webs across the bushes, or leaves trails of slime on the windowpane and mouse droppings on the sill. Or fabricates mists suspended like wreathes across the sky, opaque and milky as frogspawn in places, but filmy enough when backlit by the moon as to appear almost granular, like a loose collection of glistening, water-swelled spheres too buoyant to fall to the ground.

And we are strangers to sleep as well. Even those of us lucky enough to get it. We have an inkling of the work that sleep achieves — rest, repair, renewal, memory-fixing — and the way it takes a sonar sounding of our unconscious minds. But because this work takes place invisibly, shrouded in darkness, while we ourselves, submerged beneath our own delta waves — trapped inside a deeper darkness of our own making — are unable to witness it, we can never fully apprehend its purpose.

As the cultural historian Eluned Summers-Bremner re-minds us, 'sleep's benefits are gained at the price of our not knowing them'.

It follows that the payment that sleep exacts from us, in relieving us of consciousness, is trust.

The ancients understood far better than we do the ne-cessity of being alive to the mysteries of darkness in order to find enlightenment. The earliest Greek oracles were 'shrines to night'. Ancient heroes who wished to see things for what they really were had to pass through underworlds, or they dwelled in caves; sometimes, like Oedipus, they could see clearly (or more deeply, which is to say with insight) only once they had been blinded. After Athena blinds Tiresias for spying on her when she is naked, she gives him the gift of augury. And let's not forget the seer Phineus, who *chooses* blindness over sight. In each case truth, not light, is the source of illu-mination for the darkened seer.

In ancient Egypt, seekers after spiritual guidance could spend a night in incubation, which was a special in-stitutionalised sleep undertaken in the temples of the gods precisely in order to descry meaning in the dark. There these supplicants lay, on consecrated ground, like human lightning rods, hoping to receive messages and revelations that only the priests could interpret.

In incubation the sleeper enters a liminal realm, where the permeability of dreams allows both divine and demonic elements from the world beyond to visit the dreamer in this world. Incubation, in other words, involves crossing a threshold, replete with all the dangers of trespass that attend those much sought-after 'inner awakenings' that stand as symbols for the attainment of higher knowledge.

When my child was small her Canadian grandfather gave her a Cree Indian dreamcatcher, a spindly contraption made of thin twigs of willow, loosely braided into a hoop and hung with colourful feathers and beads and with rainbow threads crisscrossing here and there. It resembled a giant dangly earring. Zzz and I pinned it to the shelf above her bed, hoping that it would catch good dreams and channel wonder and delight directly into her sleeping head.

All these years later when I walk into her bedroom and chance upon the dreamcatcher I am moved by its talismanic qualities. Ritually, I touch the feathers, finger the cotton threads. I marvel that something so simple should channel the mysteries of the universe. Like the ancient Egyptians, the Cree Indians know that dream-seeking is an art, because what you are really seeking is the understanding that lies on the other side of the dream. The dream is just the trafficker.

There is something so peaceful about the dreamcatcher, its circular oneness, its effortless contiguity, that it seems an apt metaphor for the becalmed mind, a mind empty of worry — a darkened void across which tufts of feathery fluff or light-spun dust motes gently drift, signifying nothing. This image is the very opposite of the multi-pronged fidget spinner that comes to mind when I attempt to visualise the loud and boozy party train of senseless thought that careens across my own night-waking mind.

Perhaps one of the lessons I can take from my insomnia is that its interest lies less in what it is that we see when we are wide awake at night, prickling with longing and with an enervating need to hunt down truth, than in *how* we see. It is about paying attention to what lies at the peripheries of our being, or just across the border: or, if we can bear to look, in the abyss, where Hesiod's 'origins and boundaries of everything' are juxtaposed.

When Freud wrote about the way the conscious and unconscious minds trade insights, he, too, was attempting to fathom this matter of how we see, exposing its mechanisms, but also the way that seeing, by necessity, incorporates blind spots. What Freud says is that during the day we 'drive shafts' into our fresh chains of thought and these shafts make contact with 'dream-thoughts'. This is how day and night fertilise each other. This is how creativity is born.

It cheers me to note that because psychoanalysis works to excavate the brain's nocturnal effusions and then drag them into the light, it is essentially an insomniac practice. Perhaps that is why I am drawn to it.

If I think on how driving shafts between different thoughts can link them up imaginatively, or cross-pollinate them, or juxtapose them, invariably I arrive at the idea of collage. Dreams are collage-like. The way we grasp things is collage-like: the mind gathering in material from the outermost reaches of the senses and fusing it together into definite shapes. And writing, too, is a kind of collage, insofar as it involves a constant interaction, a millisecond-by-millisecond calibration between processing the ideas we receive and acting on those received ideas. Writing holds input and output, contemplation and invention in dynamic tension.

In a slim and most elegant appreciation of the artist Joseph Cornell (a book that is itself written in fragments), Charles Simic suggests that the collage technique that Cornell, artist, curator, scavenger, made so inimitably his own — 'that art of reassembling fragments of pre-existing images in such a way as to form a new image' — is the most important innovation of twentieth-century art. Found objects, chance creations, ready-mades: all abolish the separation between art and life. 'The commonplace is miraculous if rightly seen,' he writes.

I am inclined to agree, because the commonplace — rightly seen — is composite, contingent, unique. At best, it is transcendent.

In 1839, Henry David Thoreau witnessed just such a commonplace miracle, at the top of Saddleback Mountain in Massachusetts. Thoreau had climbed the mountain's steep and wooded slope in twilight, so there was no chance of getting down again before night fell, and so he slept on the summit. Bedding down on rocky ground at the base of the Williams College observatory, he built a fire, read scraps of newspaper, slept fitfully under some wooden boards, and in the morning he saw God.

As he describes it himself, at daybreak he discovered 'an ocean of mist' risen level with the base of the tower that 'shut out every vestige of the earth, while I was left floating on this fragment of the wreck of a world, on my carved plank in cloudland'. As the light increased, a shining new landscape revealed itself, for there was not a chink in the mist through which Massachusetts, or Vermont, or New York could be seen. Instead: 'All around beneath me was spread for a hundred miles on every side, as far as the eye could reach, an undulating country of clouds answering in the varied swell of its surface to the terrestrial world it veiled. It was such a country as we might see in dreams, with all the delights of paradise. There were immense snowy pastures, apparently smooth-shaven and firm, and shady vales between the vaporous mountains.' This newborn world of white bore no 'substance of impurity, no spot nor stain', while the earth beneath it had become 'such a flitting thing of light and shadows as the clouds had been before'.

Says Thoreau: 'I found myself a dweller in the dazzling hills of Aurora.' It was both miracle and privilege. To be in the 'very path of the Sun's chariot, and sprinkled with its dewy dust, enjoying the benignant smile, and near at hand the far-darting glances of the god' was at once aggrandising and humbling. It made him sorry for the earth's inhabitants below, only ever able to see the 'dark and shadowy under-side of heaven's pavement'.

Thoreau's everyday miracle was a chance occurrence. But it was also the product of a willingness to look at the world at a tilt. Which propensity, in turn, might be the key to unlocking the artistic mind, since where you choose to place the magnifying lens gifts you your particular vision: the oblique take, the hewing close to the margins, the subverting of norms, the tunneling down beneath surface appearances. And this skew, this tilt, is what collage teaches us too.

Collages are scattergun, random, associative. But they are also curated, controlled, and generative. Like Freud's driving shafts, they remind us that the *how* of everyday seeing is just as important as the *what*. Not least, they draw our attention to seams. It is for these reasons that whether based on visual juxtapositions or literary ones (I am thinking of William Burroughs's cut-ups and fold-ins, for example), collages have epistemological worth.

I think that love makes composites out of reality just as effectively. It fits people together, folds their lives one inside the other, reshapes our intimate worlds.

In my own composite existence, Zzz is the New World, forward-looking and thrusting, and I am Europa, full of the old anxieties and guilt. He is organised and prag-matic, whereas I dither and brood; he is inventive, I careworn. Where he is instrumental, I search out the layers beneath the layers of life's myriad layers. We are day and night to each other. We accommodate each other. We are complementary.

The French philosopher Jean-Luc Nancy conjures up these mirrored relations very well in interrogating the

meaning of sleep, when he writes of 'the sleeper hud-
dled inside the waker' and 'the waker circling inside the
sleeper'. They are enfolded together like lovers. This is
what I want to communicate to Zzz, that his essence is
enfolded within me.

I have long believed that mindfulness has its limita-
tions. It overvalues the present moment and neglects
the way the human mind wants to knit together past
and future, lived experience and speculation, so creating conditions for narrative thinking or autobiograph-
ical orienteering. With its resolute and faithful focus
on a single object of thought, or on doing away with
thought altogether, mindfulness is about as edifying as
praying to a toilet roll.

When I think about mindfulness, I cannot rid my
head of the stock image of a shiny-headed monk. Of
Far Eastern origin and saffron-robed, he is seated with
his legs knotted into a lotus, hands quietly folded. It is
an image of absolute stillness. The monk is both in this
world (there is substance and solidity to him: he is as
well fed and well tended as a healthy shrub) and yet, at
the same time, he is above the world, utterly immune
to its everyday cares. He looks as if he has been sitting

like this forever, with his eyes closed and his shoulders slightly stooped, his features — unfurrowed brow, the merest trace of a smile — expressing an exquisite peace.

This monk is the very picture of enlightenment as a kind of majestic imperturbability. When I imagine the inside of his head, I see a one-stringed instrument: pluck it and it sounds a single note, pure, unwavering, everlasting — in perfect tune with what the Zen master Thich Nhat Hanh, in a poem called 'Looking for Each Other', terms the 'one-pointed mind'.

Do I find this vision of complete contentment attractive? Yes, and also no. However much I am drawn to Buddhism's idealisation of enlightened peace, I cannot help worrying about how closely that peace appears to resemble a glorious blankness. As if the highest possible state of mind we can aspire to is the preternaturally still one that finds its homely parallel in checking out. As if attaining meditative nirvana were tantamount to a good spring clean. As if wonder had come full circle to meet stupefaction. As if transcendence meant — merely — to overcome.

I have come to the conclusion that mindfulness is much like tidying the house. It is focused and satisfying in concentrated spurts, but it lacks a direction of travel. It seeks to keep things as they are. It leaves the world unchanged.

Not like mind wandering. Which is how the mind entertains itself when it arrives at the limits of boredom. Or how it behaves, skipping, inattentive, when it is lit up in the darkness of night or, in more fruitful guise, when we dream by the light of day. Mind wandering free-associates and innovates. It overreaches wildly and pulls you along, eager in its wake. It is fleet and light and connective. It opens doors and pushes thoughts through colourful prisms. It noodles, trips, and blusters. And it roams: respecting no boundaries, it transgresses. Perhaps this is something the conscious mind can take from insomnia.

My own little sailing ship through time, my family of three wanderers, appears to have made an unspoken pact to disrupt borders. So it seems, at any rate. While I fudge and fumble my way through the hours, muddling up and stepping over night and day, Zzz journeys back and forth across the Atlantic, detonating cultural bombshells in each nation's backyard. In his newfound revolutionary zeal, he cannot help himself. Our teen-ager, meanwhile, has discovered the fertile borderlands between one gender and another and declared herself expatriate.

I still yearn for the replenishment provided by sleep. I yearn for the saving limit to sanity that lies beyond consciousness's end. All the same, I want to be sensible of the act of border crossing. I don't want to slip un-knowingly from being into nothing, but to be party to the drift and transgression, and alive to the excitement and danger that entails. It is a knife-edge business, that is for sure. And it demands that I embrace uncertainty.

I used to think that Penelope was emblematic of this border-crossing bravery. And she is. But perhaps a bet-ter representative still can be found in the heroism of Scheherazade — fabled princess of the night, her intel-ligence primed by darkness. Whereas Penelope's chal-lenge is to find a way to simply endure (the emptiness of the passing years, but also the inscrutable darkness of uncertainty and abandonment), in *The Arabian Nights* Scheherazade steps up to an altogether bigger chal-lenge, and takes on time itself.

You know the story. The Persian king is on some genocidal mission to deplete his land of womankind. Every night he beds a new virgin, but then in an act of vengeance against the infidelity of his former wife he has his new love beheaded at dawn. In Scheherazade, who volunteers herself for this deadly succession, he more than meets his match. Each night Scheherazade eases the king into sleep by spinning a marvellous new tale, and each night she leaves it unfinished in order that the now-captivated king, eager to know how the tale will end, is obliged to spare her life. Night upon night, for a thousand and one nights, she spins her stories, until the king of Middle Persia concedes defeat and marries her. (By this time they have also managed to have several children together.)

Where Penelope has her cloth, the making and unmaking of which stands as a symbol for hope, Scheherazade fills night's dread blankness with another kind of weaving. She unspools a train of dramatically colourful tales, drawing them from the distaff of her own inventive mind, and she thwarts the death sentence scheduled to arrive each dawn by suspending narrative succession. Her tactic is genius. She messes with the diurnal cycle and inserts disruption where there ought to be continuity. In this way, she masters time.

The only drawback is that Scheherazade is insomniac — and must be so in order to live. Sleep would literally be the death of her.

In alchemy there is a term for bringing something out of nothing. Specifically for bringing the philosopher's stone out of the various ingredients (who knows what? — lizard tails, hobnail boots, chicken blood, base metals) mixed inside the alchemist's crucible. That term is *nigredo*, meaning 'the blackening', and it describes the putrefaction of the *prima materia*. Nigredo is said to be 'blacker than the blackest black'. When it manifests itself you cannot believe anything good can come out of it. But just as putrefaction precedes purification, so nigredo gives way to *albedo*, or the birth of light.

Carl Jung spent long years elaborating the underlying psychological meanings of alchemy, the dark art that he understood as a symbolic language for the process of individuation — which itself is a kind of awakening, is it not? Jung took nigredo to refer to the importance of shadow work, which is the labour of understanding what you project onto others and, more important, becoming aware of your own darkness.

It takes a restless spirit to thrive on the anti-hypnotic aspects of night, to resist the lull and pull of sleep and to work instead towards becoming dark-adapted.

A restless spirit like Nikolai Astrup. Astrup is the early twentieth-century Norwegian painter renowned for his colour-saturated, quasi-primitivist paintings of rural Jølster—the sparsely populated region of western Norway that was his childhood home, and to which he returned as a young man, jaded by his studies in Olso, Berlin, and Paris, where he had felt paralysed by the influence of other (he thought better) painters. Restored to his rural paradise, he remained there until his early death at forty-seven. In Jølster, Astrup painted the dramatic landscape of mountain villages and fjords obsessively, mostly by night, producing an oeuvre of haunting paintings. He captures the glacial sheen of lake water bathed in moonlight, fields of yellow marigolds oddly radiant in the dark, and shadowy haystacks that resemble hunched and furtive humans. Everywhere Astrup's crepuscular palette succeeds in rendering the familiar strange, yet also strangely magical.

Astrup was a lifelong asthmatic for whom each night was an insomniac gauntlet of nightmares and a choking struggle for air. He habitually slept half-upright in a chair in the hall, his head slumped to his chest, only to wake in fits of 'choking seizures'. More often, he simply got up and prowled outdoors. In letters to his friend Per Kramer, Astrup hints at how he busied himself by the light of the moon, planting trees and mulching their roots with fresh soil, fishing for trout in the lake, fixing his radio, or walking through the empty town, where he took study notes on the green of the spruce trees and the quality of the light and long shadows.

I feel a strange kinship with this peculiar painter, so unlike me in every way, impossibly tall and thin, with a parson's stoop and a child-catcher's pointy nose. I warm to the way that night made a metaphysician of him.

His subject, as befits his art, was colour and mood. Astrup became fixated by the almost supernatural way that colours morphed in the dark. Blues and greys acquired a silvery intensity. Greens deepened, whites were dulled, while darkness itself became a property that arose from tangible things, like trees and stones: the moonlit sky, for its part, shone. As one scholar has remarked, Astrup understood that 'the dark allows nature to glow with its own mysterious light'. Here was a study that Astrup judged worthy of a lifetime of effort, and he indentured himself to its pursuit.

But what of my own restlessless? Where might it take me, and what kind of dedication will it demand?

The honest answer is that I don't rightly know. But when I think on the question I keep returning in my mind to that visit to Buscot Park and to what Edward Burne-Jones was trying to do with his soporific paintings.

Yet how soporific were they, in fact? In the Faringdon family an apocryphal tale survives of how Burne-Jones had been quite insistent when the paintings were installed that they be exhibited in northern light. He didn't want direct sunlight from the south falling on them, but light that had been reflected off the sky. Such light, known as 'grey' light, was the kind he worked by in his studio, since it was more faithful than direct sunlight. (Even today Kodak produces a grey card for photographers as a way of getting perfect renditions of colour and tone.) He also stipulated that the saloon at Buscot Park should be mutely lit with hanging lamps to create an air of mystery and expectation. Burne-

Jones wanted viewers to spend proper spells of time in front of the Briar Rose paintings, to encounter them in a demi-gloom that forced them to engage in a mode of seeing that called for discernment. The more their eyes grew dark-adapted, the more of the work they would eventually see — more colour, more detail, more nuance — leading to a layered understanding such as Keats might have had in mind when he praised 'slow time'.

There is plenty of nuance to catch: multiple allusions to time and eternity, for starters, scattered throughout the paintings. An hourglass whose sand has ceased to flow. A sundial that faces away from the sun. And there are peacock and swastika motifs, symbolising immortality and time's infinity, woven into the decorative features of the princess's bower. All are coded reminders that in this enchanted realm time has come to a halt. But then, along a different register, in two of the paintings there lurk tiny, half-hidden windows, painted into the background, beyond which the real world — the waking world — goes on, fully illuminated and fully alive. So there is a beating heart in the frame, after all. But what was Burne-Jones trying to tell us?

In 1890, coinciding with the paintings' popular unveiling, *Punch* magazine published a piquant cartoon. Titled 'The Legend of the Briar-Root', it purported to be a 'companion subject' to the Briar Rose series, and in each of its four scrawnily drawn frames the same set of characters are slumped, lost to an opium sleep. A couplet echoing William Morris's verse about the sleeping handmaids trills, 'The Maidens thought the pipe to fill: They smoked, and now they all lie still.' The cartoon's wicked humour (which relies on its audience knowing that the hard, woody roots of the Briar Rose were commonly carved into tobacco pipes) implies that Beauty's enchanted sleep is actually a drugged one. This was the age not just of the rest cure, but also of chemical anaesthesia and laudanum treatments — an age when slumbering women of one kind or another came to symbolise the malaise of an entire society enslaved by material culture, closed off from imagination and living off its nerves.

This is the world Burne-Jones wanted to shake up. And who can blame him?

The briar rose, or dog rose, is seldom cultivated domestically, as a garden plant, because it is spiky and woody and aggressive, but also because unlike other, tamer varietals, it flowers for only two weeks of the year. During its brief bloom the plant is garlanded with delicate pink flowers, cherished for their sweet apple-like fragrance and much-prized in wedding bouquets. Look again at Burne-Jones's canvases and you see that his briars are exploding with blossom. Everywhere you look, there is a profusion of flowers, flicks and flecks of pink, confetti-like and joyous. But is the plant flowering (waking up!) because the prince has arrived to claim his bride? Or is it perpetually flowering, as a reminder of the world beyond, holding out its eternal light?

Perhaps the suggestion is that there is an awakening nestling or curled up within every enchantment, prefigured somehow, presaging a revelation.

Burne-Jones's unconscious mind may well have seeded meanings in his work that resonate far further afield than he intended. But I like to think the process of dark adaptation that he wanted viewers to experience *was* planned. Because this way a trap is set, so that each viewer, however fleetingly, might experience an awakening of their own, which, if taken to heart, might allow them to wake up to themselves and their potential;

to rally and organise and agitate for revolution; to embrace uncertainty and welcome change.

This is what I wish to effect in my own life, the better to discern the flicks and flecks of pink so casually strewn across my fields of vision and experience. I want to flip disruption and affliction into opportunity, and puncture the darkness with stabs of light.

This is the song of insomnia, and I shall sing it.

Sources

INDISPENSABLE SOURCES

Elisabeth Bronfen, *Night Passages: Philosophy, Literature and Film* (Columbia University Press, New York, 2013).

Eluned Summers-Bremner, *Insomnia: A Cultural History* (Reaktion Books, London, 2008).

DEEPER SOURCES

Gwyneth Lewis, *Sunbathing in the Rain: A Cheerful Book About Depression* (Flamingo, London, 2002).

Tom McCarthy, *Satin Island* (Alfred A. Knopf, New York, 2015).

Maggie Nelson, *Bluets* (Wave Books, Seattle, 2009).

Charles Simic, *Dime-Store Alchemy* (Ecco Press, Hopewell, N.J., 1992).

OTHER SOURCES

Gaston Bachelard, *The Poetics of Space* (1958). New edition (Beacon Press, New York, 1992).

Gennady Barabtarlo, ed., *Insomniac Dreams: Experiments with Time by Vladimir Nabokov* (Princeton University Press, Princeton, N.J., 2017).

A. Marshall Barr, Thomas B. Boulton, and David J. Wilkinson, eds., *Essays on the History of Anaesthesia*, International Congress and Symposium Series 213 (Royal Society of Medicine Press, London, 1996).

Matilda Bathurst, 'Northern Light'. Review of Nikolai Astrup exhibition at Dulwich Picture Gallery, 2016, *Apollo Magazine*, vol. 640, no. 1, pp. 196–97.

Charlotte Beradt, *The Third Reich of Dreams: The Nightmares of a Nation, 1933–1939* (1966), translated by Adriane Gottwald (Aquarian Press, London, 1985).

Elizabeth Bishop, 'Crusoe in England', from *Complete Poems*, with a new introduction by Tom Paulin (Chatto & Windus, London, 2004), pp. 162–66.

Robin Blackburn, *The Making of New World Slavery: From the Baroque to the Modern, 1492–1800* (Verso, London and New York, 1997).

Claes Blum, *Studies in the Dream-Book of Artemidorus* (Almqvist and Wiksell, Uppsala, Sweden, 1936).

Roberto Bolaño, 'The Worm', in *The Romantic Dogs*, translated by Laura Healy (New Directions, New York, 2008).

Georgiana Burne-Jones, *Memorials of Edward Burne-Jones*, with a new introduction by John Christian, vol. 2, 1868–1898 (Lund Humphries, London, 1993).

Blake Butler, *Nothing: A Portrait of Insomnia* (Harper Perennial, New York, 2011).

Susan P. Casteras, *Images of Victorian Womanhood in English Art* (Fairleigh Dickinson University Press, London and Toronto, 1987).

Nancy Cervetti, *S. Weir Mitchell, 1829–1914: Philadelphia's Literary Physician* (Penn State University Press, University Park, 2012).

William Gervase Clarence-Smith and Steven Topik, eds., *The Global Coffee Economy in Africa, Asia, and Latin America, 1500–1989* (Cambridge University Press, New York, 2003).

Stephen Cushman, 'Make the Bed', in *Cussing Lesson* (Louisiana State University Press, Baton Rouge, 2002), p. 22.

Cynthia J. Davis, *Charlotte Perkins Gilman: A Biography* (Stanford University Press, Stanford, Calif., 2010).

Galya Diment, 'Nabokov and Epilepsy', *Times Liter-*

ary Supplement, August 3, 2016, www.the-tls.co.uk
/articles/public/sudden-sunburst.

Roger Ekirch, *At Day's Close: A History of Nighttime*
(W. W. Norton, New York, 2005).

Sigmund Freud, *The Complete Introductory Lectures on
Psychoanalysis*, translated and edited by James Stra-
chey (George Allen & Unwin, London, 1971).

Charlotte Perkins Gilman, *The Living of Charlotte Perkins Gilman: An Autobiography* (1935), introduction
by Ann J. Lane (University of Wisconsin Press, Mad-
ison, 1990).

Charlotte Perkins Gilman, *The Diaries of Charlotte
Perkins Gilman*, vol. 1 (1879–1887), vol. 2 (1890–1935),
ed. Denise D. Knight (University of Virginia Press,
Charlottesville, 1994).

Gayle Greene, *Insomniac* (University of California
Press, Berkeley, Los Angeles, and London, 2008).

Sasha Handley, *Sleep in Early Modern England* (Yale
University Press, New Haven, 2016).

Homer's Odyssey, ed. Lillian E. Doherty, Oxford Read-
ings in Classical Studies (Oxford University Press,
Oxford and New York, 2009).

J. Donald Hughes, 'Dream Interpretation in Ancient
Civilisations', *Dreaming,* vol. 10, no. 1 (2000), pp. 7–18.

Carsten Jensen, 'Life's Detours: A Portrait of Nickolai
Astrup as a Comic-Strip Character', in *Nikolai Astrup, Dream-Images*, translated by John Irons and

Francesca M. Nichols (exhibition catalogue, Gl. Holtegaard) (Narayana Press, Copenhagen, 2010), pp. 114–19.

Maria Konnikova, 'Why Can't We Fall Asleep?' *The New Yorker*, July 7, 2015, followed by 'The Work We Do While We Sleep' and 'The Walking Dead', also in July 2015.

Peretz Lavie, *The Enchanted World of Sleep*, translated by Anthony Berris (Yale University Press, New Haven and London, 1996).

Anne Leonard, *The Tragic Muse: Art and Emotion, 1700–1900* (Smart Museum of Art, University of Chicago Press, 2011).

Penelope A. Lewis, *The Secret World of Sleep: The Surprising Science of the Mind at Rest* (Palgrave Macmillan, London, 2013).

Øystein Loge, *Nikolai Astrup: Betrothed to Nature*, translated by Francesca M. Nichols (Det Norske Samlaget and DnB NOR Savings Bank Foundation, Oslo, 2010).

Rowland Manthorpe, 'Mind-Wandering: The Rise of an Anti-mindfulness Movement', *The Long+Short*, December 10, 2015, thelongandshort.org.

Fiona McCarthy, *The Last Pre-Raphaelite: Edward Burne-Jones and the Victorian Imagination* (Faber & Faber, London, 2011).

Sidney Mintz, *Sweetness and Power: The Place of Sugar in Modern History* (Viking Press, New York, 1985).

Rubin Naiman, 'Falling for Sleep', *Aeon*, July 11, 2016.

Jean-Luc Nancy, *The Fall of Sleep*, translated by Charlotte Mandell (Fordham University Press, New York, 2009).

Sanjida O'Connell, *Sugar: The Grass That Changed the World* (Virgin Books, London, 2004).

Mary Oliver, *New and Selected Poems, Volume One* (Beacon Press, Boston, 1992), p. 181.

Jeremy Over, 'It's Alright, Students, Not to Write: What Ron Padgett's Poetry Can Teach Us', *Writing in Education*, vol. 71, NAWE Conference Collection 2016 (2), pp. 39–44.

Ruth Padel, *In and Out of the Mind: Greek Images of the Tragic Self* (Princeton University Press, Princeton, N.J., 1992).

Ruth Padel, *Whom Gods Destroy: Elements of Greek and Tragic Madness* (Princeton University Press, Princeton, N.J., 1995).

Cristina Pascu-Tulbure, 'Burne-Jones's Briar Rose: New Contexts', *English: Journal of the English Association*, vol. 61, no. 233, pp. 151–75.

S. F. R. Price, 'The Future of Dreams: From Freud to Artemidorus', *Past and Present*, vol. 113 (1986), pp. 3–37.

David K. Randall, *Dreamland: Adventures in the Strange Science of Sleep* (W. W. Norton, New York, 2013).

Jennifer Ratner-Rosenhagen, 'American Dreaming 3.0', *Aeon*, May 25, 2017.

Benjamin Reiss, *Wild Nights: How Taming Sleep Created Our Restless World* (Basic Books, New York, 2017).

Rumi, *Selected Poems* (Penguin Classics, London, 2004).

Oliver Sacks, *Awakenings* (1973; new rev. ed., Harper Perennial, New York, 1990, and Picador, London, 1991).

Elaine Showalter, *Hystories: Hysterical Epidemics and Modern Culture* (Columbia University Press, New York, and Picador, London, 1997).

Lisa Russ Spaar, ed., *Acquainted with the Night: Insomnia Poems* (Columbia University Press, New York, 1999).

Kasia Szpakowska, 'Nightmares in Ancient Egypt', in *Études d'archéologie et d'histoire ancienne*, Collection de l'Université de Strasbourg, Actes des journées d'étude de l'UMR 7044 (Strasbourg, November 2007), pp. 21–39.

Henry David Thoreau, *A Week on the Concord and Merrimack Rivers*, ed. Carl F. Hovde, William L. Howarth, and Elizabeth Hall Witherell, with a new introduction by John McPhee (Princeton University Press, Princeton, N.J., 2004).

Marina Warner, *From the Beast to the Blonde: On Fairy Tales and Their Tellers* (Chatto & Windus, London, 1994).

Stephen Wildman and John Christian, *Edward Burne-Jones: Victorian Artist-Dreamer*, with essays by Alan

Crawford and Laurence des Cars (Metropolitan Museum of Art, New York, 1998).

Emily Wilson, *The Odyssey* by Homer, a new translation (W. W. Norton, New York, 1917).

John J. Winkler, *The Constraints of Desire: The Anthropology of Sex and Gender in Ancient Greece* (Routledge, New York and London, 1990).

Lawrence Wright, *Warm and Snug: The History of the Bed* (Routledge & Kegan Paul, London, 1962).

Acknowledgements

Here's to those who put tempting things in my path as soon I mentioned I was working on this book, or introduced me to a poem in another context that came good here, or pointed me to a scholarly work I would have never found otherwise. For these gifts and favours I thank Heather Dyer, Anne Goldgar, Julia Copus, Wendy Monkhouse, Tina Pepler, Emma Crichton Miller, Jeremy Over, Joanne Limberg, Jude Cook, Michael Marmur, Nigel Warburton, Sally Davies, Scott Weightman, and Samantha Ellis.

At Buscot Park in Oxfordshire, Roger Vlitos was welcoming and generous in sharing his enthusiasm for and knowledge of Edward Burne-Jones. It was a privilege to be allowed to see the paintings in situ and to hear juicy anecdotes about Burne-Jones's life and work. At the Kode Galleries in Bergen, Sigurd Sandmo and Tove Hausbø went beyond the call of duty and enthusiastically dug into the archives on my behalf to unearth interesting notes and letters from the Nikolai Astrup papers (now being translated into English).

Thank you to my fellow insomniacs for making the sleep clinic bearable; to Tina Pepler and Anna Barker, with whom I teach creative writing to academics — I hope they will approve my spinning of some of what we do into this book. Thank you to Brigid Hains: no one could wish for a more insightful and careful first reader. Thanks to Rebecca Carter and Emma Parry for championing this book from the get-go; to the inspirational Philip Gwyn Jones at Scribe and Pat Strachan at Catapult, who fully bought into my experiment, and to Sarah Braybrooke and Erin Kottke, publicity geniuses both.

Permissions for reprinting poetry were granted from various quarters. I have quoted lines from Stephen Cushman's poem 'Make the Bed' with the kind permission of the author. The stanza from 'Insomnia' by Marina Tsvetaeva that appears as an epigraph here was translated by Elaine Feinstein and appears in *Bride of Ice* (2009), copyright Elaine Feinstein. The lines are reprinted here with permission from Carcanet Press Limited, Manchester, UK. The excerpt from 'Crusoe in England' is from *Poems* by Elizabeth

Bishop, copyright © 2011 by the Alice H. Methfessel Trust; Publisher's Note and compilation copyright © 2011 by Farrar, Straus and Giroux; reprinted by permission of Farrar, Straus and Giroux. The poem also appears in *Poems* by Elizabeth Bishop, published by Chatto & Windus, reproduced by permission of the Random House Group, Ltd © 2011.